The Eye
Diet

How Not To Go Blind

Dr. Christopher Maloney, N.D.

Copyright © 2018 Hygeian Publishing

All rights reserved.

ISBN-13: 978-1720599555

ISBN-10: 1720599556

DEDICATION

To the hopeless, that they may hope. To the blind, that they may see.

CONTENTS

ACKNOWLEDGMENTS

I want to thank my teachers and fellow students over the years, from high school to Harvard and NUNM. You have inspired in me the thirst for knowledge and the courage to push the limits of what is possible. Let me acknowledge and thank my optometrists for giving a blind boy the gift of sight. I want to thank my family and my patients for listening to me and trying what I suggest. You have taught me through both my failures and successes. I want to thank all my readers. You teach me every day what you need. When I get a message from one of you telling me that I've helped you, it makes me feel for a moment that I'm doing my bit for the universe.

WARNING

This book is for informational purposes only. Please don't think that I have any way of knowing what's wrong with your eyes. Do consult your eye doctor (or several) about any health conditions involving your eyes. Use this book to inform your discussion, to help you understand their treatments, and to educate yourself about your eyes. Be well, and take care of yourselves.

1 Who Needs This Book?

I did. You do if you plan to live beyond middle age and have eyes that have gotten worse in recent years. The world does, because we're seeing eye problems increase worldwide.

In this book you're going to learn how to improve your sight. No, I'm not promising to cure your eye problems. I'm not going to claim that I've cured mine. But I am going to explain how your eyes work, how to make your eyes healthier, and how to improve your ability to see. As part of that, we'll talk a little about what you should eat to help your eyes (that's the diet part). But mostly we're going to completely change how you see your eyes.

My own story starts as an eye conformist, getting glasses early on and wearing them religiously exactly as prescribed. As I reached midlife, I could no longer see. I've been nearsighted (can't see far away) since junior high. But now I couldn't read supermarket labels without taking my glasses off. It made me a candidate for another pair of glasses, reading glasses for seeing better close up. Or I could get my glasses combined into bifocals, or even trifocals, for reading, near vision, and seeing into the distance. I tried the newest tri-focal glasses my optometrist happily made me, spending a month as nauseous as a seasick passenger on stormy seas. There weren't any other options. So I went looking for this book.

I wanted a book to help me improve my eyes just a little so I could read labels again. According to my optometrist my goal was impossible, but I'm stubborn. I wasn't trying to go out and get rid of my glasses. As a descendent of people with glasses, I had the genes. I knew I would always wear glasses. But I wanted to regain a little bit of my recently lost sight. My optometrist shrugged and made me another appointment in six months. It was pretty clear he knew I'd be back.

And I may be. I've spent my life in glasses, so for me to expect not to need stronger ones over time may be the height of foolishness.

But I can say that in three weeks of minimal effort (about five minutes a day) I don't have to take my glasses off to read labels any more. Sure, that could fade. But I think it's worthwhile to pass on how I did it. I also want to tell you everything I've learned about the eyes in the process.

Changing the way your eyes function isn't just in your eyes. It means changing your assumptions about how your eyes should function. So we're going to learn how the eye works in simple language. We're going to make you rethink what you know about the eye.

As we go along, please question everything I say as well as everything you've been taught before. I'm going to provide you with lots of medical articles that support what I say (all those tiny roman endnote letters sprinkled through the book will each bring you to a medical article). Ask your eye doctors for the same research about anything they tell you. If there isn't a study behind what they say, it's what they've been taught, and may not be accurate. I know, because as a doctor I was taught a lot of misinformation about the eye.

If you feel that the new information seems radical, please realize that I wrote this book based on what I found in the medical literature (all eye doctor reviewed and approved). I started off researching just how I could improve my own eyesight just a little. What I found has made me question everything I was taught as a doctor about the eyes.

Even though what I'm going to say may change how you view your eyes, knowing this new information does not mean you will regain any eyesight. Applying the knowledge on a daily basis in your own life is the only thing that will produce changes.

With actual change in mind, I wrote this book as simply as I could. We will be using words like ball and balloon rather than long medical terms like posterior chamber and vitreous body. By the end you won't be able to pass a quiz on the parts of the eye. But I hope you'll understand enough about the eye to help you to see better.

Again, I cannot promise that you will regain eyesight. Some people may improve. Others may require surgery. If some of you improve your eyes to a point where you no longer need glasses, I will be thrilled. If that happens, I fully credit you with doing all the work. All I can do is point you in the right direction.

Much of this book asks you to approach your sight differently. Please, do not mistake me for an eye guru who demands you discard your glasses. I've read enough fanatics to recognize that compassionate, slow improvement is far better for long term health. So I'm a firm believer in glasses if you need them, but I'm not a believer in accepting progressive vision loss as inevitable.

For those of you who require evidence of my personal success before reading further, I will say that in one minute on the second day of my personal experimentation I was able to improve my near reading. By the second week, I could read better using my weaker eye. In the third week, I no longer needed to remove my glasses to read labels at the grocery store. I'm editing the printed pages of this book without my glasses, something that would have been impossible a little over a month ago.

But I ask that you not rely on my personal experience, because yours will vary widely from mine. I am purposefully writing and publishing this book while I continue this journey myself, so that you realize we are all sharing the same struggle to see. I will share my own journey alongside medical studies to give you a better sense of what you might expect yourself.

The future of my eyesight rests in my own hands. As does yours. Let's begin.

2 Isn't Eyesight Genetic?

MY PERSONAL HISTORY

I was born to be blind. My great-grandparents had glasses. My grandparents had glasses. My parents had glasses. So, of course, I would need glasses. I knew my eyesight would be bad.

Once, as a child, my mother told me that unless I read in better light I would need glasses. I told her I was going to need glasses anyway because she had them and so did my dad. Then I told her it was good, I wanted glasses. For me having glasses meant you were now an adult. It was a rite of passage like learning to drive.

But I didn't know when to ask for glasses. By the eighth grade, my eyesight was so bad that even in the front row of the classroom I could no longer read the blackboard.

For the previous two years I'd been surviving by pushing against the outside of my left eyelid to see the board. The best way to visualize this is that I was pushing my eye into a slant, removing all the slack in my eyelid and literally altering the length of my left eye slightly. Doing so changed my eye length, bringing the blackboard into sharp focus for a few seconds at a time so I could write down my homework assignments with my right hand. I didn't understand why it worked, I just had figured it out while bored one day in class. Trying to prop my eyelids open with my fingers resulted in an improvement in my sight.

EXERCISE: EYE TUG

To do what I did, place your fingers on the outside edges of your eyes and pull gently (never hurt your eyes) back toward your ears. If you pull too hard, your eyes will blur. But a gentle tug will slightly alter your focus. Fine tuning the tug may improve your unaided vision enough to read a distant sign. This technique has helped me often if my glasses aren't handy.

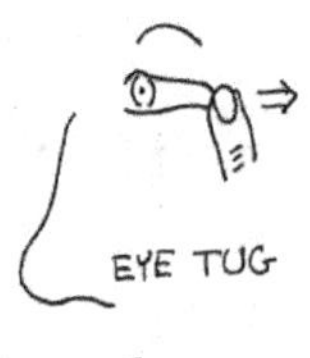

I finally asked for glasses when I got a teacher who wrote on the blackboard in such tiny letters I couldn't see even from the front row. Sitting with one finger constantly pushing my eyelid back was considered disruptive.

My first pair of glasses were immense. I wanted to be able to see as much as possible, so I chose oversized frames. The result was a pair of glasses so heavy they slid continually down my oily teenage nose. For decades after I discovered sticky silicon nose pads, I still pushed up my glasses as a nervous habit.

Something strange happened when I got glasses. For the first few years, my eyes got worse. Then my eyes stabilized to almost the same prescription for decades. Because I am an unbelievable packrat, I still have my eighth grade glasses. My left eye has deteriorated slightly, but my right eye can still use my eighth grade glasses. So it is basically the same prescription thirty years later. For my left eye, I can still see 20/20 using old lenses I got in college. So my vision has been stable for at least two decades.

Now that I've hit my late forties, again my vision is deteriorating (which makes me suspicious that something hormonal is happening). But now it's my near vision, my sacred reading space, that is being intruded on.

I never minded having glasses for far vision. The frames kept the harsh world at a distance. I was safe from the hurts of the world behind my personal window frames. When I tried contacts, I found them personally frightening. Everything was too clear, too close. The contacts were also painful, as I have too much of what my optometrist calls "eye dandruff," which I can only assume is bits of my eyelid skin getting onto the surface of my eyeball. But the real reason I never looked into eye surgery is because I liked wearing glasses as my personal distancing devices.

Now, as I begin middle age, my reading ability is threatened. My greatest and oldest escape from the world is under attack. Instead of the satisfaction I felt when I got my first glasses, joining the ranks of my adult relatives, I now fear the loss of my sight for the first time. The promise my old optometrists made to me that, as a nearsighted person I'd never need my glasses to read, has been broken. So for the first time in my life I've truly questioned this strange world of vision.

But how can I expect my eyesight to be better if my lineage decrees my eyes will start badly and worsen over time?

ARE WE BORN TO BE BLIND?

If you look back at classic medical eye studies, one of the first in the 1920's was a study of identical twins who shared difficulties with eyesight. So we've known eyesight was related to genetics since at least the 1920s.[i] (Here's the first of those endnotes if you want to look up the twin study and read it yourself.) Another twin study was done as recently as 2017. The medical news trumpeted, "Identical twins have identical vision, down to the smallest detail."[ii] These identical twins had identical eyes and eye problems, even after fifty years of living separate lives. The author of the 2017 study even claims that the eyes of identical twins are so similar they see the distant stars exactly the same way.

Case closed, right? Eyesight is clearly entirely genetic. Yes, there's the problem that identical twins don't necessarily represent the rest of the population. But that feels like nitpicking, because the twins show us that genetics are king when it comes to the eyes. I guess this is going to be a very short book. We can wrap things up and wish everyone the best of luck. Go out and blame your parents if, like the cartoon character Mr. Magoo, you bump into things as you get older.

But what's funny about the twin studies is that the studies aren't as conclusive as the authors would like. In the 2017 study, the results showed only 70% of the identical twins' eyesight was due to genetics.[iii] That's similar, but not identical. Another recent study of identical twins found that, as they got older, they had significantly different eyeglass prescriptions.[iv] So environmental factors clearly play a significant role in how well even identical twins see. Once you move away from identical twins, fraternal twins have significantly different eyesight. So eyesight is not determined only by genetics, even in twins.

Still, isn't eyesight deterioration mostly genetic? We all know families with glasses tend to have children with glasses, right? Yes, but those families also share habits, diet, and lifestyles. Just because mom and dad have glasses doesn't mean genetics determine whether or not little Joey or Susie gets glasses.

What I found when I started looking at the genetics of eyesight was very strange. Yes, some rare eye diseases are truly genetic. But the common eye illnesses are multifactorial, which means that my genes only play a small part in how my eyes function.[v]

A SILENT PANDEMIC

I still expected to find that eyesight is mostly genetic, occurring at roughly the same rate generation after generation in populations around the world.

Instead I found a silent and largely ignored pandemic of rapid eye deterioration occurring on a global level. If this was any other disease, it would have foundations, marches, and monthly updates from our public health experts. It makes our annual flu pandemics look like nothing because, unlike recovering from the flu, no one is recovering their lost sight. Once you're blind, you stay blind.

But this was the first I'd heard about the pandemic, and I spend my life reading medical literature for both work and fun. (I know, sick, right?)

The first study about the pandemic I saw talked about nearsightedness showing up in eighty percent of Asian young people.[vi] I couldn't believe the rate could be that high. I thought the author must be making it up or playing games with statistics to alarm the public.

So I questioned that number. But other major medical articles cited similar statistics.[vii] The World Health Organization (WHO) is concerned enough about the problem to commission a study on how to prevent further nearsightedness (myopia).[viii]

Let's be clear. The WHO isn't worried about a little fuzzy distance viewing, they are worried about extreme nearsightedness that can lead to blindness.

We're talking about globally occurring, rapidly increasing nearsightedness so bad it's causing retinal detachment, cataracts, glaucoma, and macular degeneration. All of the common eye diseases of old age are visiting these young people far earlier than expected. It's gotten so bad, doctors are using lifelong drug prescriptions to try and prevent further worsening of young people's nearsightedness.[ix]

In the U.S., the numbers aren't as bad as Asia. The number of nearsighted people in the U.S. has just jumped from 25% to 40% since the 1970s. It's nothing like the jump from 18% of South Koreans in 1955 to 96% of South Korean twenty-year-olds today.[x] That's an extreme jump in a genetically stable population.

Then I started looking at the projections of increasing eyesight loss for the future. The problem of severe nearsightedness is going to get worse all over the world. Experts estimate half the planet will be nearsighted by 2050, and extreme nearsightedness will affect one in ten people.[xi]

When they say extreme nearsightedness, the experts mean near-blindness and all the common diseases that we currently associate with old age. Right now the number of people with extreme nearsightedness is only about two percent, so it's going to jump five-fold in the next thirty years. Not double or triple. We will have five times as many people with near-blindness.

That cheery futuristic 2050 report shows even more rapidly progressive increases in nearsightedness worldwide since the year 2000. So something we're doing in the last ten years has dramatically worsened the situation.

The genetics of the world haven't changed, but our lifestyles have. Specifically, we've added a lot more near viewing and long hours in front of our screens. There's a term for it, called Computer Vision Syndrome, which includes the common symptoms of eye strain, burning eyes, and eye fatigue.[xii]

> *"The symptoms of too much screen time can include:*
> *(1) eye fatigue;*
> *(2) eye pain;*
> *(3) eye heaviness;*
> *(4) unfocused eye;*
> *(5) blurred vision;*
> *(6) double vision;*
> *(7) burning sensation;*
> *(8) eye dryness;*
> *(9) excess tearing;*
> *(10) foreign body sensation;*
> *(11) itching;*
> *(12) spasm of eyelid;*
> *(13) sensitivity to bright light;*
> *(14) different color sensation, and*
> *(15) headache.[xiii]"*

Could other things be affecting our global eyesight? Of course. But it's hard to argue for other lifestyle factors impacting eyesight as much as increasing screen time (and the corresponding lack of outside distance-viewing time). Nearsightedness only affects one in twenty East Africans, but it affects half of Asians living in high-income economies.[xiv] If you look at most other health markers, high income Asians have it better than East Africans, who are genetically prone to having a higher pressure in their eyes (glaucoma). But these same high income Asians are outpacing East Africans ten to one for nearsightedness.

BEYOND GENETICS

Now, I'm not saying genetics don't play any role in eyesight. It's possible to have both a genetic cause and a lifestyle cause for eyesight loss. But the rapid and dramatic loss of eyesight in young people worldwide coincides with the increase in screen time and near vision work. It does not coincide with any genetic shifts or mass migrations. The genetic influence on nearsightedness for South Koreans might be as high as 18%, but that leaves the other 78% of their current vision loss as entirely environmental. So instead of thinking that genetics could explain all of our eyesight loss, we need to start looking farther into how we got where we are.

Remember, I'm not the one going out on a limb and saying we have a pandemic of vision loss. We're talking about an analysis and review of over a hundred eye studies published by global experts who say we now have a quarter of the world's population with nearsightedness. That amount is going to double to half the world's population being nearsighted by 2050. They estimate nearly five billion people will be nearsighted. Of that group, they fear that one in five may be so severely nearsighted they could be blind. That could be one billion nearly blind people by 2050.[xv] It's pretty alarming, and even more alarming that it hasn't made the nightly news.

HINDSIGHT

In retrospect, (hindsight always being 20/20), I learned about the rising epidemic of nearsightedness years ago. Back in 2000 I had the privilege of living in Singapore for a year, and I learned during my visit about the Singaporean industrial and technical revolution.

Since gaining freedom in 1965, Singapore moved from being a backwater to being one of the "Asian Tiger" economies of the 1990's. Not bad for a tiny little island thirty miles across.

But Singaporeans knew even back when I was there that their rapid development had come at the cost of higher levels of nearsightedness.[xvi] It seemed like a small price to pay to become a developed nation basically overnight. But they've since documented that nearsightedness doubled (in the same genetic population) during the transition from developing to developed country.[xvii] At the time I was there, I thought it made sense, since rush hour in Singapore is 7 am and 9 pm six days a week (they work all day and only get Sundays off).

But I never really connected their national experience with my own experience or my own eyes. Sure, Singaporean eyes were affected by moving inside and staring at screens all day, but that had nothing to do with my genetic inheritance and my eyes. Besides, if there was anything I could do personally, I'm sure my optometrist would have told me. He didn't, and only recently have I started to ask myself why. But before we understand why my optometrist didn't think anything could improve my eyes, we need to know more about what an eye is and how we see.

3 What Is An Eye?

Since I've become concerned about what is happening in my eyes, I've started looking at the eye itself. It's a wonderful, complicated organ that we don't fully understand even now. But I'll keep things simple.

Let's learn about the eye. I know, the next thing I'm supposed to do is put in this book a graphic of the side of an eye, with lots of labeled bits that are supposed to help you picture the eye better. And we all know that what you'll be left with is confusion. By tomorrow, you won't know an image of the eye from a map of Albania. "Is that an eye or Albania?" you'll ask me.

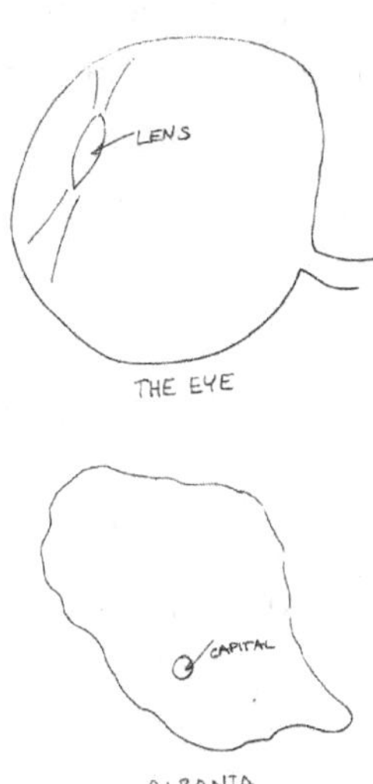

Basically all most people get from an eye graphic is a balloon with a magnifying glass lens at one side and a long nerve coming out the other. There are dozens of these online, and they don't tell us much that we can use.

If anything, eye graphics make the eye seem complex, alien, and so confusing we don't think we can ever understand it. Honestly, even in medical school it doesn't get much less confusing. Now that I've read the experts, there's a lot about the eye (including how pressure builds up inside the eye) that we don't totally understand and experts still argue about. When we look at a map of the eye it's still a bit like looking at an old map of the world. At the edge of what we knew for certain, the old mapmakers used to write, "Here be monsters." That's what a map of the eye still feels like. Don't look too close, because it is still confusing even to the experts.

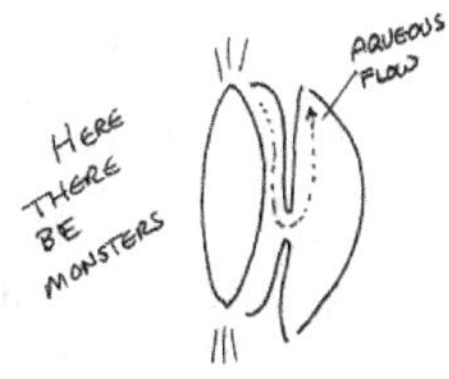

So we'll use a different kind of visual aid. If you're reading this, you have eyes. Blink for me. Those are your eyelashes and eyelids coming up and down. Squeeze your eyelids tight and then open them a few times. What you feel squeezing are the muscles around your eyes. Look at your nose with both eyes, then up and out at the outer corners of your eyebrows (extra points if you can look out at both eyebrows at once). Now look up, down, left, and right. Finally, roll your eyes for me (if you aren't already from how silly this is), all around in a circle. Congratulations! You've now found all of the six outer muscles of your eye. Not only that, you now know how they all work.

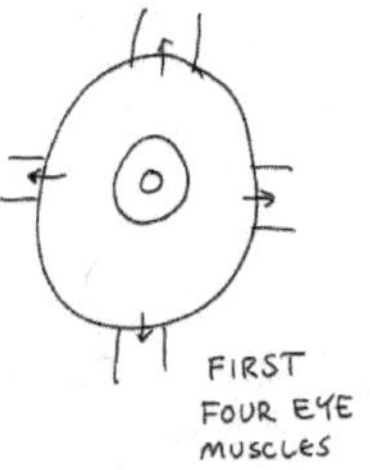

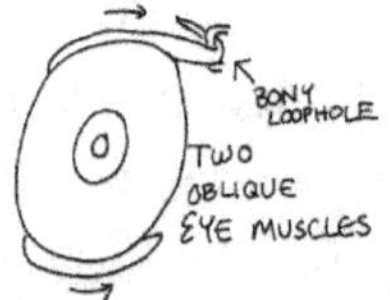

Let's learn about the surface of the eye. Squeeze your eyes tight and open them a few times. You should feel more moisture on the surface of your eye. These are tears. They come from tear glands under your upper outer eyelids. When they drain, they drain into the tear ducts at the lower inside of your eyes. Those tear ducts drain into your nose, which is why when you cry your nose runs (at least some of it, the rest is snot). When they are on the surface of your eye, those tears provide your eyes with all the nutrition they need. Most of the tears are water, but that water is mixed in with a little bit of oil. You've got oil glands all along the upper eyelid. If they don't work, you can wet your eyes all day long with saline solution and they won't stay moist.

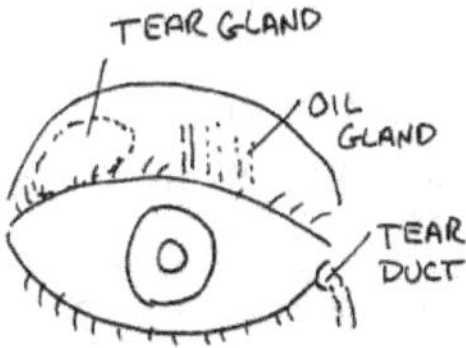

If you look at this page, what you shouldn't see are blood vessels clouding your view. Your eyes are clear at the front of where you see. The front "skin" of your eye has no blood vessels. It gets its oxygen directly from the air, dissolved in your tears, during the day. At night the tears give it oxygen as well as nutrition. So the surface of your eyes are really dependent on tears. How about another eye roll to give your eyes a breather?

The inside of the eye is a little more tricky to understand. Look at this page, then far away. Pick up your finger, look at your finger, then far away. What you just did, with or without glasses, is to tighten the tiny ciliary muscles in the front of your eye to change how you see. The muscles do this by making the lens and front of your eye thicker or thinner.

Inside the front bit of your eye, in an area smaller than the thickness of your little fingernail, your eye muscles were tightening and relaxing. When you look far away, they relax and the front gets thinner. When you look closely, they tighten and the lens and the front of your eye get thicker.

These tiny eye muscles are what we tighten all day long when we look at things close to us. The tiny muscles are pretty strong because they have the most energy production of any muscles in your body. But they are muscles, the same as your arm or leg muscles.

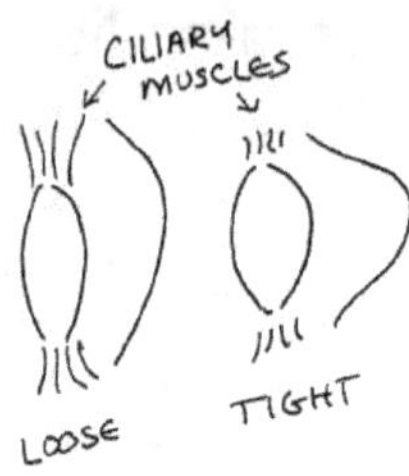

Now think with me about how often we look at a distant horizon these days compared to a near screen. Yep, our eyes spend almost all their day tensed to see closer and never gaze at that far off horizon to relax. At night, just because your eyes are closed doesn't mean they are relaxed. Anyone who has seen a dog, cat, or child sleep knows the eyes are seeing dreams as if they are real. So don't expect your eyes to undo a day's strain at night just because your eyelids are closed.

All of that muscle strain is at the front of the eye where the lens is, which focuses the light for the back of your eye. So all that eye tension exists in an area roughly the size of your pinkie finger nail. The rest of your eye is there to receive the focused light and translate it into sight.

The back of your eye is a fascinating place. Look at this book (paper or electronic). Now close your eyes and see the remaining image of the book inside your eye. Maybe you just see the outline of a reading device, or maybe the outline of the book. You may see the outlines of the letters or the white space around them. What you're seeing is the residue of viewing the page happening inside your eye. When you open your eyes to see, tiny particles of light (photons) from the screen or page bounce into your eye and trigger different reactions in the back of your eye. It's not important to know all the pieces of the back of the eye that make this possible (rods, cones, etc.) What's important is that you can see the results of anything you do to the back of your eye very quickly. Look at a bright light, and you'll immediately get a very bright residue when you close your eyes. That residue gradually repairs itself, so the color of the light will change from white to another color as the back of your eye repairs first some parts and then other parts of your vision. You can literally see this happening while you wait. The eye is repairing itself that fast.

It's also really important to realize how much of what you receive into your eye you don't pay attention to. That light residue is happening all the time. It's like a constant silent fireworks display happening every time you blink. But you ignore it when you read these words. Your brain is wired directly to your eye. It's constantly interpreting all the light coming in, filtering out 99% of it, and "telling" your conscious brain about the 1% it thinks is important. If I do something like write "konichiwa," your brain decides that's a garbage word, or a greeting in Japanese. Your eye is receiving tons of light bouncing off everything in your surroundings, and yet for the moment all you are aware of is that one word.

We can show that all the extra information you receive from all that light is actually distracting to your eye seeing well. Please find a piece of paper and a pin, needle, or thumbtack (a pen or sharp pencil will do). Yes, you can use a page of this book as the paper if you must, but you might be happier if you use a bit of scrap paper.

Now make a pinhole in the paper, take off your glasses, (contact wearers may want to wait until the end of the day) and hold the pinhole up to your eye. If you look through the pinhole and close your other eye, you should be able to read the words more clearly. (OK, you can put the glasses back on now.) The pinhole limits the amount of light particles (photons) coming into your eye. It gives you a thin stream of relevant light, light you can use to read the letters on the page. Yes, using a pinhole can instantly improve your eyesight by shutting out the distraction of all the other light (and images) coming into your eyes. Pinhole eyeglasses can be created cheaply, and might help the millions of people who currently do not have access to prescription eyeglasses.

HOW THE EYE CHANGES FOCUS

Now we've seen a single beam of light coming into the eye. Let's talk for a minute about how the eye deals with lots of light. Clearly it does a really good job of making clear images for us out of chaos.

When you think of light coming into your eyes, think of it like waves of light crashing into a narrowing harbor up onto a narrowing beach between two rocky cliffs. As ocean waves hit narrow cliffs, they slow down. What's left of the wave gets funneled into a smaller and smaller area, so that the wave that laps the back of the beach is a tiny little wave. That tiny little wave touches the back of the beach at a focal point.

For light, hitting our eye is like hitting a narrowing cliff. The light gets narrower and narrower the farther it goes into the eye. Part of the reason for this is that the light is passing from the air into the ball of water that is our eye. If you've ever looked through a glass of water, everything beyond the glass is distorted. The light in the air has been bent and slowed by passing through the glass of water the same way an ocean wave might be bent and slowed by hitting narrow cliffs. So waves of light coming straight at the eye are going to bend and narrow toward a single focal point at the back of the eye.

CLOSE FOCUS

If we wanted to make crashing waves of light get very narrow very quickly, we'd need very thick cliffs that could narrow the wave very rapidly. In the eye, we need a thicker lens.

The muscles of our eye tighten around the eye lens, forcing it to get thicker and narrow light more. So light coming from very close can be bent only by a great deal of effort from the muscles of the eye until it is narrow enough for us to see it at one focal point.

As you can imagine, looking at things very close all day long forces the eye to work very hard tightening on that lens. The eye will try to make things easier for itself to see things up close by lengthening the eye over time. A longer eye requires less focus and means less work for the eye muscles.

But a longer eye can cause problems for seeing far away. Imagine having a faraway wave hitting those thicker cliffs with a longer beach. The faraway, weaker wave doesn't even reach the back of the beach. In the same way, the longer eye is too long to see well far away. The light wave fades out before the back of the eye and isn't in focus. People with longer eyes can see things up close just fine (even easier than normal folks), but they can't see things are away. We call these people nearsighted (myopia) because they can see things up close but not far away.

What if the waves of light are too strong for the eye? If ocean waves are so strong they come pouring through and the cliffs aren't narrow enough to slow the flood, the beach will be washed out. In the same way, if the eye can't tighten enough to narrow the light coming from very close, a person can't see things up close no matter how hard they try. We call people who can't see things up close farsighted (presbyopia), because they can only see things far away.

But wait, you can have both! As we get older, our lenses stop being as flexible (just like the rest of us). They can no longer flex and get thick enough to narrow the light and see things up close. As your eye gets less flexible, you may find yourself reading with your arm farther and farther from your eyes. You're trying to get the light wave to come from far enough away to read the words. Your eye lens can't narrow the light from up close even if you have longer, nearsighted eyes.

If you've been nearsighted your whole life because of your longer eyes, you can also lose your ability to tighten your muscles around the lens. So now you can't see anything either far away or up close. There is an area a few feet in front of you that is reasonably clear, but you need help for seeing both near and far.

EYE CRUTCHES

If you're farsighted, seeing things up close is relatively easy. You just need another lens like the one in your eye, an extra helper to help narrow the light more. These are magnifying lenses (they make your eyes look bigger, and the letters on the page look bigger). If you want to know what kind of lenses are in a pair of glasses, just hold them up and see if they make nearby things bigger. Those are magnifying lenses. They can be found in any supermarket or drugstore in various strengths and are very inexpensive. People generally buy them for reading and have multiple pairs. If anything, getting these eye crutches for the eye is too easy because using them incorrectly may not be best for the eyes (more on that later).

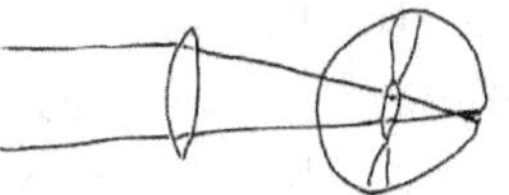

If you're nearsighted, seeing far away clearly is a little more tricky. If you have a longer eye and can only see things up close, you need a crutch that will bend the light outward for you. Basically, you need to add power to the waves of light coming in, giving them extra push to get to the back of your eye. So your eyeglass crutch widens the waves instead of making them narrower. The lens you need to add will make your own eye's lens seem thinner. Light will be bent outward by the glasses, then back in by your too-thick eye lens to reach the back of your too-long eye. When you look through the glasses of a nearsighted person, their eyes will seem smaller, because the lens makes it appear like their eyes are farther away.

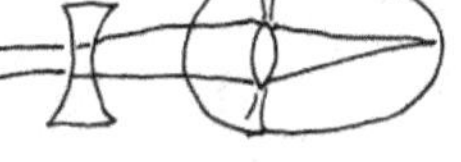

So what if you don't really need glasses and get them anyway? What happens when you give a healthy eye an extra lens to look through? If that lens is a magnifying lens, like the reading glasses farsighted people need, the change will be more narrowing of light. The healthy eye will want to get shorter from end-to-end to reach the new, closer focal point. To get shorter, the back of the eye will get thicker.

What happens if you do the opposite, giving a healthy eye a lens for a nearsighted person that bends light outward? The extra lens will put the focal point "behind" the back of the eye. So the back of the eye will become thinner, and the eye will start to grow longer if it can.

Since the eyes work together, not only will the wrong lens affect the eye looking through it, it will affect the growth of the other eye as well (at least in chickens).[xviii]

So the same eye crutches that allow a nearsighted or farsighted person to see better (the lens of the glasses) can also contribute to the worsening of that person's sight? Yes, if the eyeglasses are too strong, they can make the eyes worse. Perhaps a good reason for not using another person's reading glasses, and for getting the lowest possible eyeglass prescription you need.

How fast does the back of your eye significantly change? Put the wrong eyeglass lenses on school-aged child, and the back of her eye will get thinner or thicker within two hours. It can also correct itself again rapidly if she is later given the right prescription.[xix] In healthy people the back of the eye is constantly changing, affected by blood flow, age, and time of day.[xx] So the back of your eye is constantly trying to correct and heal itself.

FOCUSING ON THE FRONT OF YOUR EYE

Right underneath the surface of your eye is the area that focuses the light. It's an area that these days spends almost all its time under tension. It's also the area where fluid pressure can build up, until it becomes a problem that can affect how well you see (glaucoma). Diseases like glaucoma are happening in that tiny, pinkie fingernail-sized area of the front of your eye, when the fluid gets trapped or blocked. If the fluid builds up, the front of your eye gets thicker. A thicker eye means you can't focus well. Physicists estimate that our eye lens only does about 20% of the light bending in our eye. The front of the eye and the back of the eye do the rest.[xxi] (The front does most of it.[xxii]) So having fluid collect in your eye can render your lens useless and make you blind. One of the things that moves that fluid most effectively is heat.

Let's take a moment to stop reading and put our palms over our eyes for five breaths. My hands are cold (it's winter here in Maine) but just having the darkness and the increasing warmth of my palms feels restful. I am literally altering the flow at the front of my eye. Maybe not significantly enough for a lab technician's measurement, but significantly enough that I notice it. We need to know how much we can effect the front of our eyes, because something as simple as a cup of coffee can increase eye pressure (though the coffee flavonoids also help eye health)[xxiii] while a cup of tea may decrease eye pressure.[xxiv]

If you want to check and see how much pressure is in your eyes right now, close your eyes and lay the pads of your fingers very gently over the closed lids (without any pain, please, we're not trying to cause any discomfort). Back when doctors lacked modern machinery, they used their fingers and described an eye with too much pressure (glaucoma) as being "rock hard." For most of us, the feeling of the front of our closed eyes is soft and giving. Again, please don't cause yourself any pain as you gently explore the closed eyelid. My fingers are sensitive enough to tell that one of my eyes (the more nearsighted one) is slightly longer from end-to-end (or just protrudes more) than the other one. Both feel about the same softness. Both eyes feel closer to my nose than to the outside bones of my eye socket. Don't be concerned with not being able to find things. The goal is just to learn about how your eyes feel.

When I have my finger pads placed very gently on my closed eyelids and I move my eyes around, I can feel my eyes moving. It feels to me like my eyes move a lot more when I look up than when I look down. Looking left doesn't require as much effort as looking right. I realize that I do look down far more than up, and I look left when I drive far more often than I look right to check my mirrors. So it makes sense that my eye has gotten better at doing these things. I may have done enough of one activity that my eye muscles have moved my eye around in its socket to make it easier for me to do that thing more easily.

Hopefully even though we don't now have a lot of long words to go with your eye, you have a better sense of how your eye works. Since you'll be the one checking on yourself every day to see if anything in this book is helpful or has changed your eye, it's a good idea for you to have some idea of what you're working with. Your experience with your eye on a daily basis is the best way we have for telling if your activities on a given day helped or harmed your eyes.

4 What Is Sight?

Why should we talk about seeing separately from the eye? Because what your eye takes in and what you see are very different things.

Your eye is a light-consuming organ. It is made to take in any and all light. As soon as your eye is open, (and even when it's closed through the red of your eyelids) light from the outside streams into the eye. The eye bends that light with the front of the eye to concentrate it, and it receives all that light with the back of the eye. If you think about your eye's purpose, it is to collect light particles from wherever it can and to focus them into a tight beam for our brains.

Our eyes take in everything around us, all the time they are open. There are, right now, literally thousands of bits of information coming into your eye. The colors of the room, the position of your hands, your position in space, other people or animals in the room, changes in the amount of light in the room, where your furniture is. The list goes on and on. Until I brought it up, chances are good that you weren't aware of most of those things. Your eyes viewed them, but you didn't see them. They were background noise, like advertisements or people passing in a car. Unless you are focused on them, they don't enter into your experience of conscious sight.

Our expectations that sight is the same as "what we see with our eyes" isn't remotely true. There is a famous video of a gorilla walking through a basketball game. If you distract people by making them count the number of basketball passes in that video, half of them won't see the gorilla at all.[xxv] It's called inattentive blindness, and it's what most of us do, most of the time, with most of our world. We only see that tiny sliver of the world we want to focus on and pay attention to. Today that area may be more and more often limited to a glowing screen the size of your open palm (more on that later).

But knowing that we're ignoring the majority of what our eyes take in has an enormously beneficial side. It means we can see much better than we do, even if our eyes are getting worse. I know, it seems nonsensical to say we can see better if our eyes are worse at seeing, but bear with me.

Let's start with the standard explanation of how the eye works. The front of the eye tightens, thickening itself, to focus on something. That focus brings light to the back of the eye. Like a magnifying glass, that light shines on a single point in the back of the eye (the fovea). Officially that single point is the only place in the eye that can have perfect vision. So your total sight is determined by that single point. If that point is messed up, your vision is messed up.

But, even without advanced degrees in optics, we know this isn't true. Take your thumb and put it out in front of you at arm's length. The average area of the clear part of your vision (the central fovea) should be roughly twice the size of your thumb.[xxvi] OK, now look off at a wall or something in the distance. Do you only see two thumb's width clearly? No, you see a full wall (hopefully) with a range of clarity. If you let your eyes relax to not focus on one spot, what you see is the full panorama of what is around you, not limited by that tiny central area of maximum clarity. Sure, you can focus intensely on one tiny spot on the wall (is that a spider or a paint chip?) but you see the whole room with varying levels of clarity.

Even if we were to limit ourselves to that tiny center point of our vision, it's not a single spot. It is tiny, roughly the size of the colored end of a pointer pin or a round sprinkle on a cupcake. But that means that you have more than one point of ideal focus. You may not be using it, but you have many more spots where you have perfect vision.

As we move out from that center point, you still have pretty clear vision. It's not perfect, but close enough to do most of your daily activities. If you allow your eyes to relax and take in this whole page of text, chances are pretty good that you can recognize some of the words that are not exactly where you're looking. The "As" at the beginning of this paragraph may still be visible and recognizable even when you're looking down here. If not, let your gaze relax until you can see the whole page again. Allowing your vision to "soft focus" can allow you to see much larger areas of text.

Wait, if something is visible and recognizable, isn't that the same as seeing it clearly? No, because it's not quite as clear as if you look directly at it. But if we're talking about something like text, being able to recognize text is the whole point. No one (except the font lovers out there) cares about the exact shape of the "N" at the beginning of this sentence. The rest of us see it as an "N" and move on. We don't need fully functioning central points to read if we train ourselves to read with our peripheral vision.

Yes, train ourselves to read. While the central focal point

of the eye takes up a tiny area in the eye, most of the part of the brain dedicated to sight is focused on processing information from that tiny area.

If we started tomorrow to turn our heads to the left until we could barely see this page, none of our central point could see the words. Only our peripheral vision (which is blurrier) would be used. But over time our brains would learn to interpret that blurrier information. We might need bigger print, or even a magnifying glass at first, but if we started now over time we could train ourselves to read using the peripheral parts of our vision.

We don't necessarily need to go to that extreme. It's enough to realize that we habitually use one tiny area to see which is part of a much larger, very clear area three times its size. Simply allowing ourselves to experiment, using slightly different ways to see things, means that over time we can become more flexible about seeing things with different parts of our central focusing area. Having that flexibility means that if something happens to our single habitual point we are using we can move to another point quickly and easily without losing any clarity. It's like practicing writing with your other hand. We hope we don't have to rely on it, but it's great to have the option.

Right now, with your lenses on, turn your head from side to side. The lenses you are wearing only "perfectly" correct your eyes at their center. At the edges things get more blurry. If you take off your lenses and move your head around, looking up or down at the letters, you will find certain angles of your sight are more clear or less clear. Your eye is not a smooth, perfect surface. Like the rest of our bodies, our eyes have variation across their surfaces. For me, looking up without my glasses is much clearer than looking down. But looking down with my glasses on is clearer than looking straight forward. As I've become more aware of how I'm seeing, I realize how limited my eye habits have become. Just turning my head slightly feels strange and distracting. I've become used to viewing my world exactly the same way, in exactly the same position, for decades.

Remember, your eye is viewing much more than you're seeing. Rather than straining to keep seeing the same exact way, open yourself up to seeing things slightly differently and you may see better. The information is there, you're just not open to receiving it. Making the decision to be open to seeing things differently is the first step to improving your sight (and your life).

5 Why Treat Eyes Separately?

Let's start with the big picture. It doesn't make a lot of sense to think about the eyes as separate organs from the rest of the body. They share the body's blood supply and need similar nutrition, requiring a great deal of both to do the job of seeing.

But we do think of the eyes differently from the rest of the body. The eyes have different doctors, who give different prescriptions, and the doctors who treat the eye have different expectations than other doctors.

The difference doesn't seem dramatic until you think about how we treat the eyes in another medical context. Let's use the example of how we treat a broken arm.

THE EYE AS AN ARM

If you went in to your emergency room with a broken arm, the ER doctor would set you up with a cast. Six weeks later, the cast comes off. Your arm will be weaker from lack of use, and you'll need to exercise it to bring it up to speed. But it would be completely healed in a few months.

Imagine if you went in to the ER with a broken arm, and

they treated your arm like eye doctors (optometrists) treat your eyes.

Instead of fixing the break, the ER doctors take lots of detailed measurements of your arm. Using those measurements and a new 3D printer right there in the ER, they print you up a very expensive, form-fitting cast made specifically for you. It fits your arm perfectly and you are pretty impressed.

"When does this come off?" You ask your doctor.

"Oh, it will never come off," says your ER doctor. "We expect your arm strength will change over time, so you'll need to have the cast fitted again every year. But if you wear it all the time, this cast should be all you need to function again. Isn't it a great color? They just came out with this new style."

"Wait," you say, "You mean I have this cast for life?"

Your ER doctor nods. "You'll need to wear this cast until you need a stronger one. As people age, many of us need two casts, one for heavy lifting and one for desk work." He rolls up his sleeve, and you can see he's wearing two casts himself, a big one and a smaller one underneath. "I've got the newest bi-use cast that does both functions. There are even new tri-use casts. But don't worry about that right now. Just enjoy your new cast!" He waves his two casts at you as he leaves.

Hopefully if you had that experience with an ER doctor you'd leave angry and confused. After a few days, you'd seek a second opinion. Why? Because somewhere you heard that arms can get better. Arms can heal. You've even seen people get their arm casts off. So you know you don't need to wear an arm cast for the rest of your life. You go looking for a second opinion.

But with the eyes, there are no second opinions. Every optometrist, every doctor of ophthalmology, will tell you the same story. (There are a few exceptions, and we'll get to those in a bit.) The eyes get old, they stop working right, and you need corrective lenses for the rest of your life. It's likely you'll even need eye surgery if you live long enough. Eventually your eyes fail you. At best, you can expect slow deterioration. At worst, you go blind.

"Will anything help?" you ask your third eye doctor.

"Not really. Diet and lifestyle have no effect," he says.

"What about eye exercises?" you ask as the doctor's hand is on the door.

"You could try. But studies show nothing like that works. It's just your genetics," he shrugs.

How strange that we see eyes so differently from the rest of the body. Let's go back in time to see how this became the "normal" way to treat the eyes.

EYE CARE THROUGH HISTORY

To go back to the beginning, we have to go way, way back. People have been trying to correct poor eyesight for a very long time, from the time of the Egyptians (with their football-style makeup under their eyes to reduce sun glare) on to the present day.

It's possible that the Greeks used curved clear stones to try and see better. Glasses were likely first created in India or China and made their way to Europe.

In the western world, the first glasses were discussed in the 13th century. The people who made these first glasses were glassblowers, not doctors.

So for centuries the profession of optometry was the profession of making and dispensing glasses. It had nothing to do with examining the body. The makers of glasses did not need medical degrees. Ben Franklin famously even created bifocals for himself. So there was no medical degree, just an apprenticeship with an older optometrist to create and dispense eyewear.

THE RISE OF OPTOMETRY

The profession of optometry did not arrive at its present lofty medical position easily. Optometrists began to be prosecuted at the end of the 19th century for practicing medicine without licenses. In 1895, optician Charles Prentice was threatened with jail for charging for an eye exam.[xxvii] He was an optometrist, trained as an apprentice under his father, following in his father's trade. His father had practiced the same way in the same city since 1847.

The year after his trial, Charles Prentice started an association to support legalizing his profession. This association eventually became the current American Optometric Association (AOA) (as proudly related on the professional timeline on the AOA website).[xxviii] When it first began, the AOA did not require members to be opticians. Any and all manufacturers of optical devices could be members. A set of professional standards for the AOA wasn't enacted until 1935.

It seems like standards might have been needed. In 1937 Richard Riis published *Optometry on Trial* in Reader's Digest, claiming the profession simply existed to sell eyeglasses.[xxix] Riis did a bit of early investigative journalism, bringing the same patients to different optometrists. Healthy patients who did not need glasses all got glasses of various strengths, and no optometrist agreed on the same prescription for any patient. More troubling, sick patients with severe eye issues weren't referred to other medical doctors for further care.

The AOA struck back at this negative article with a book of its own and a call for greater professional unity. Even so, the degree of Optometrist was not recognized until 1951. In 1966, optometrists won an antitrust lawsuit against the American Medical Association, who had up to that point blocked its medical members from associating with or referring to optometrists.

The common practice of optometrists over the last century was to fill their prescriptions for patient glasses only in-house, not allowing patients to shop elsewhere. Enough people complained that in 1978 the Federal Trade Commission finally issued a rule requiring that eyeglass prescriptions must be released to the patient.

Clinical practice guidelines were sent to all members of the AOA in 1994 and New Standards of Professional Conduct were adopted by the AOA in 2011.[xxx] Even today, lens prescription errors can occur after the lens is placed into different frames.[xxxi] (But prescribed glasses are still much better than ready-made lenses from a store.[xxxii])

While I love my optometrist, he still tries to sell me his eyeglasses from his own office supply. Now I understand why.

THE OPHTHALMOLOGISTS

There is another group of doctors who treat the eyes. These are surgeons, doctors specializing in the treatment of severe diseases of the eye. The first eye surgeons date back to 2250 BC. In the laws of Hammurabi an eye surgeon who failed to heal the eye he treated could lose his fingers.[xxxiii]

Despite this lengthy lineage, no organization of eye doctors existed for thousands of years. The first organization of ophthalmologists in the U.S. began in 1896, the same year the optometrists organized. So these medical doctors only bonded together to face the threat posed by the optometrists on their medical turf. The organization of ophthalmologists was formed from within the larger association of doctors who specialized in eyes, ears, noses, and throats (today's EENTs) and the two specialties did not truly separate until 1979.[xxxiv] So it can be said that there has not truly been a profession of eye doctors until very recently.

Now that we finally have a distinct group of medical professionals focusing only on the eye, we would hope that more medical research is finally taking place. But a recent analysis of one hundred and twenty-four studies on the errors of sight found only eleven of them were reliable.[xxxv] Of all the studies about the eye, the most reliable studies have been done on surgery for the eye. We still lack big, long term studies on things like which kinds of eyeglasses help eyesight more. Some studies show that, other than helping us see now, eyeglasses do nothing to slow the deterioration of the eye.[xxxvi]

THE STORY OF EYESIGHT LOSS THROUGH HISTORY

Knowing the history of eye doctors gives us insight into how we got where we are now. We can see better how we came to think about the eye as separate and different.

Back in the beginning of the profession, hundreds of years ago, there were doctors and there were people who did eyeglasses. Most people weren't sick enough to see the doctors, they just needed eyeglasses. So for the common person on the street, they got all their information about the eyes from people who sold eyeglasses.

The people who made eyeglasses didn't have degrees. They weren't doctors, they were craftsmen. Skilled craftsmen, but not interested in the rest of the body. You came to them for eyeglasses. The experience of these craftsmen was that people gradually needed stronger lenses over time. As people got older, they needed different, stronger glasses. It was a good, sustainable business model.

Craftsmen who made eyeglasses weren't in the business of figuring out why people kept needing stronger glasses. It was just part of old age. They sold eyeglasses, and they were most interested in people continuing to buy eyeglasses. Why would they rock the boat and ask questions about why people needed eyeglasses? Or if people really needed glasses at all? So the craftsmen told their customers that the eyes just get worse over time. Nothing to be done. It's probably the Gods (and later your parents') fault.

EYES VS. TEETH

Compare the attitude of ancient eyeglass craftsmen to another group of craftsmen, the traveling dentists. These fellows would go from town to town pulling teeth. Sometimes they'd leave a tooth for later, but mostly what they did was pull teeth. Their bread-and-butter relied on their customers' bodies being able to repair themselves, because nobody wants a tooth pulled if they're going to die from infection afterward. Traveling dentists told customers that when they pulled your tooth, the body would heal itself. Not just the skin, the bone of the jaw. So today's dentists, who emerged as a separate medical profession from that traveling dental tradition, depend on the body to heal itself rapidly and completely.

Today modern dentistry relies on the ability of an aging person's jaw to grow new bone around dental implants. An aging jaw to a dentist is a vibrant, healthy place that can heal itself fully. It forms permanent new bone around a metal implant strong enough to attach a fake tooth that can be used to chew hard foods day in and day out. If the body couldn't fully heal itself, much of modern dentistry could not exist.

Dentists are a good comparison to optometrists because they are a doctor that most people see when they are relatively healthy. With both dentistry and optometry, we are talking about the face. If a fake tooth is implanted into the jaw in an older person, it takes place literally an inch below where that same person's eyes are continually and progressively deteriorating, with no chance of ever improving. Yet the jaw completely heals.

The jaw is able to heal, but the eyes cannot. Dental surgeons feel comfortable doing surgery and assuming that an aging body will marshal sufficient resources to heal the surgery, keep off infection, and lay down new bone for the sake of easier chewing. Yet an inch above where the dental surgeon is working the eye is unable to heal itself after decades and allows itself to go blind. It certainly seems like a leap of faith on the part of dental surgeons.

Astute readers may have thought of one area where optometrists (or at least ophthalmologic surgeons) do trust the eye to heal fully. When eye doctors perform surgery, they assume the eye will heal fully and completely. If your ophthalmologic surgeon takes out your cataracts (another inevitable decline) and replaces your lens with a fake one, she assumes you will heal nicely and be fine in a short time.

So if you can perform surgery on the eyes and they recover fully and completely, why is it that no one is treating the underlying problem of progressive eye decline? Why aren't we preventing blindness rather than just approaching it with last minute surgery? Why, after thousands of years, are we still pulling out eye lenses like rotten teeth rather than helping the person prevent their decay in the first place?

6 Why Not Change Eye Care?

We don't do the same things we did a century ago in most areas of medicine. Large studies have shown us that much of what we thought was good for patients (like bleeding or mercury tonics) are bad. But eye care seems trapped in a time warp. Why haven't doctors tried to treat the eyes differently? The answer lies in the cautionary tale of an eye doctor heretic, Dr. William H. Bates.

WHAT'S WRONG WITH DR. BATES?

Once upon a time in the early 1900s there was an eye doctor who thought differently about how the eye functioned. Rather than saying the eye was doomed to deteriorate, Dr. William H. Bates said the eyes problems were caused by strain and fatigue. Given proper rest and exercise, the eye could repair itself. Dr. Bates came up with a series of eye exercises that he said would help patients recover, and these still exist at the alternative fringe of medicine (where I live) as the Bates Method. Why didn't the Bates Method become the normal way eyes are treated today?

Well, according to Dr. Bates' New York Times obituary, he was a lunatic. By the time of his death in 1931, Bates had become a medical outcast. His obituary openly talks about him as a wandering madman prone to periods of paralyzing anxiety.[xxxvii] Yet at one point he had been a respected eye doctor, so it's hard to completely ignore Bates.

To promote his ideas about the eye, Dr. Bates' wrote and self-published an eye care book. His 1920 *Perfect Sight Without Glasses* is now in the public domain.[xxxviii] (Later versions are still under copyright.)

Recall that Bates was publishing at the same time that the first twin studies were coming out saying that all sight loss is genetic. Bates was fighting an uphill battle, arguing with all comers. Dr. Bates not only said that all his colleagues were wrong, he also called them idiots to their faces and in print.

Bates' book was not shy about the brilliance of its author and the foolishness of his colleagues. By the ending chapter, it is clear that Bates had already lost significant prestige and position because he refused to play politics or hold his tongue. Any truth of what he found was lost to his colleagues because of the arrogant way he presented it. Rather than engaging his colleagues, Bates dismissed them.

When Dr. Bates listed the reasons for his book, it made me feel deja vu about our current situation with eyesight: "there is not only no cure... no palliatives save those optic crutches known as eyeglasses."[xxxix] A century later we're in the same situation. In what other area of medicine have we advanced so little in nearly a hundred years?

Bates continued his 1920's book by citing army statistics of worsening eyesight of soldiers in Europe and America. We now know he was seeing the beginning of the pandemic that is now finally getting the world's attention.

But at the time he seemed to be grasping at straws.

Then Bates put in his book photos of natives of various cultures squinting at the camera, claiming this proved the widespread increase in nearsightedness. The assumption that these people had vision defects and weren't simply uncomfortable with the photographer lacks credibility.

So far, there was nothing to recommend Bates' book. But then Bates made the case that his ideas were based on extensive clinical experience. He didn't set out to claim a different cause for eyesight loss, he discovered it.

> *"Examining 30,000 pairs of eyes a year at the New York Eye and Ear Infirmary and other institutions, I observed many cases in which errors of refraction either recovered spontaneously, or changed their form, and I was unable either to ignore them, or to satisfy myself with the orthodox explanations, even where such explanations were available. It seemed to me that if a statement is a truth it must always be a truth. There can be no exceptions. If errors of refraction are incurable, they should not recover, or change their form, spontaneously..."* [xl]

To test the eyes of his subjects, Dr. Bates used a retinoscope, a viewing device superior to today's Snellen chart (created in 1862)[xli] and the test lenses optometrists still use to prescribe eyeglasses. Most doctors use retinoscopes today to test for damage in the eye but not for telling how clearly the eye can see near or far objects. Dr. Bates' method was to view the eye from six feet away, a difficult task for most doctors.

Bates was so disturbed by the changing nature of his patient's eyesight he started doing both human and animal experiments.

> *"Finally, about half a dozen years ago, I undertook a*

series of observations upon the eyes of human beings and the lower animals the results of which convinced both myself and others that the lens is not a factor in accommodation, and that the adjustment necessary for vision at different distances is affected in the eye, precisely as it is in the camera, by a change in the length of the organ, this alteration being brought about by the action of the muscles on the outside of the globe." [xlii]

There are no large scale studies reproducing Bates' experiments and showing that he was wrong. But about this change in the shape of the eye, we know more now. We have much better imaging today of the inside of the functioning eye.

Bates was wrong, the lens does change in thickness as we shift from near vision to far vision. And the overall length of the eye does not change dramatically in mature adults as we try to see near or far. These errors have been pounced on by his critics as evidence that all his ideas are completely false.

But Dr. Bates gave his critics even more fuel to burn him. He told people in his book they could look at the sun. Nothing else in Dr. Bates' book makes critics as angry as his offhand remarks that staring at the sun will not make you blind (p. 187, with picture). To be fair, he says that some people do not go blind, while others do. He prefaces his remarks by citing animal studies that bright light blindness is temporary. But we are left with Dr. Bates vs. the world when it comes to looking at the sun (as anyone who saw the recent solar eclipse with welder's goggles will attest).

I do not pretend to even fathom Dr. Bates' assertion about sunlight. Yes, it is true that some people can gaze at the sun without permanent damage. Even in 1999 people watched a solar eclipse without protection, and only half of their eyes were permanently damaged.[xliii] But telling people that staring at the sun won't make you blind is like telling people jumping off the roof won't break your legs. It's sometimes true that you won't have a broken leg, but why on earth would you want to recommend it? It feels like Dr. Bates was willfully baiting his colleagues, telling them nothing they believed about the eye was true.

What Bates was getting at is a common misconception about bright light and eye damage. Even today we don't have a clear connection between bright light and permanent eye damage.[xliv] But we can see that damage can happen when very strong exposures (lasers, welding) occur.[xlv] So most of us avoid too bright sunlight because it's unpleasant and might hurt us. Bates' claim otherwise might be true for some lucky individuals, but it's not something any of us should strive for.

Of course, being me, I had to try this out myself recently. Just a quick flash of direct sun was enough to leave me with spots. They started white, went purple, then gradually faded to pink. Relaxing my eyes didn't change anything. So I'd have to join Bates' critics and "just say no" to staring at the sun.

WHY BOTHER WITH BATES?

But just because Bates was wrong about some things, arrogant about others, and guilty of poor judgment with some of his recommendations, that doesn't mean his entire framework is wrong.

The attitude of Bates and response of his colleagues recalls the unfortunate case of Dr. Semmelweis. Dr. Semmelweis was an fanatical advocate of hand washing for doctors before we knew about the existence of bacteria. Semmelweis called his colleagues irresponsible murderers for not washing their hands. We now know he was right, but that didn't stop his colleagues from committing him to an insane asylum where he was beaten to death by guards. Had he lived twenty years longer, Semmelweis would have seen his hand washing supported by Pasteur's discovery of bacteria as the cause of disease. But Semmelweis lacked patience and the wisdom to not antagonize his colleagues. It seems that Dr. Bates suffered from a similar impatience. If he had lived to the present day, Bates would at least have confirmation of the nearsighted epidemic he predicted.

Was Dr. Bates right the same way Dr. Semmelweis was? Can the eyes be fixed? I honestly don't know, though there are some intriguing case histories, a number of individuals (Grace Halloran, Aldous Huxley) who have claimed great help from reading his book.

Perhaps the most stunning case of Dr. Bates' exercises helping someone is Meir Schneider. Mr. Schneider went from being stone blind as a child to getting a driver's license without corrective lenses.[xlvi] He's made a life career promoting his version of Bates' exercises and now runs a school in California to help others.

Just having one blind man saying Bates helped him see makes all the negative commentary pale in comparison. If it worked for even a single individual, what is the harm in promoting it more broadly?

More importantly, Bates said the reason for poor eyesight was straining of the eye. He did a series of experiments where he showed that tension on the external muscles of the eye caused animal eyes to change focus. Today we know that relaxation is necessary for a fully functioning eye.[xlvii] Chronic eye tension is an issue that is now recognized as a factor in the high rates of nearsightedness.

With the mindset that Dr. Bates was not a complete lunatic, let's start again at the beginning with William H. Bates.

WHAT'S RIGHT WITH DR. BATES?

William H. Bates was an oculist (today's ophthalmologist), a full eye doctor, who was excellently trained at Cornell and Columbia. He showed all the signs of being a great New York doctor, accomplished in his field and publishing medical research. Among his other accomplishments, Bates discovered adrenaline.

The New York Times obituary fails to mention Bates' scientific work, his extensive clinical practice in several New York hospitals, or the experiments Bates did on the shape and function of the eye. It was these experiments that convinced Bates that the muscles of the eye affected sight. He documented how sight changed the shape of the eye, and came up with ways to improve sight greatly over a short period. These findings, presented to his colleagues as medical research papers, formed the basis of Bates' heresy. His colleagues thought the eye was fixed, unchangeable, and sight could not be improved the way Bates described. Since his experiments could not be refuted, Dr. Bates was presented to the world as a madman who could be disregarded entirely.

Dr. Bates claimed the lens of the eye did not change. He was wrong, the lens of the eye does get thicker and thinner, aiding in the focus of the eye.

But the lens is not the only part of the eye that shifts as we try to see. So does the entire front of the eye, the cornea.

Experts currently estimate that the eye lens provides less

than a third of our ability to see, with the front part of the eye providing the rest.[xlviii]

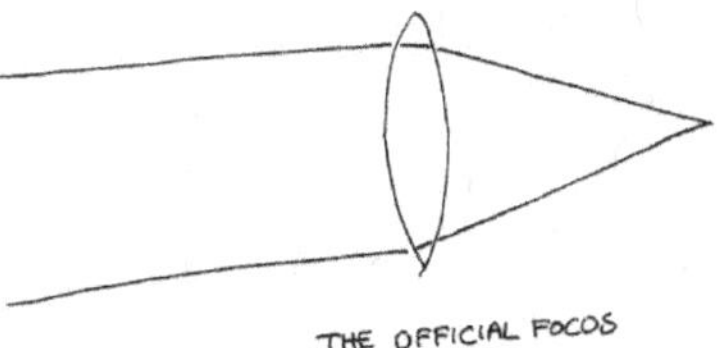

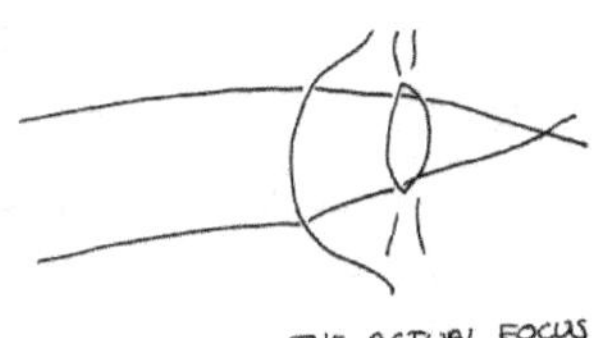

So Bates was not wrong about the eye's overall shape affecting our sight. He overlooked the effect of the lens, and he thought the entire eye changed shape. What happens instead is mostly a shift in the front of the eye, either bunching up or flattening out. Everything in the front of the eye is involved to some extent.[xlix]

Bates was right that sometimes the eye can learn to see better even without the lens. Modern researchers have documented changes in the front of the eye after cataract surgery has replaced the lens with a fixed piece of plastic. The eye still tries to accommodate, just not very well.[l]

So why did Bates think the entire eye changed shape? Part of the problem may have been that Bates wasn't limiting his views of the eyes to mature adults. In children, and especially in adolescents, the actual eye length does change over time. The longer the eye, the greater the chance of nearsightedness, and the more changeable the length of the eye. Most of this change occurs during adolescence, so most nearsightedness worsens during this time. If Bates was including young people in his experiments, he may have misjudged the change caused by adolescent growth with daily shifts in the eye.[li]

The eye can also become longer if you put it behind the wrong lenses. Guinea pigs given the wrong lens prescription had their eyes grow longer.[lii] It's also possible to use other lenses to make the eyes of other mammals grow shorter.[liii] When Bates was practicing was long before the Reader's Digest article came out about the lack of standardization in eyeglass prescriptions. Bates was seeing eyes before optometrists had established professional practice guidelines. So it is very possible he was, in fact, seeing the results of improper eyeglass prescriptions as part of his studies.

Even in young adults, there is still a slight shift in the length of the eye, something you can cause to happen in a period as short as an hour using the wrong lens prescription.[liv] If Bates' patients were wearing the wrong lenses, their eye length could have been changed.

You can also change the length of a young person's eye after exercise. The entire eye shortens as the pressure within the eye normalizes.[lv] A similar effect can be seen in young people after drinking lots of water, with a greater change in the length of the eye in nearsighted people.[lvi] So if Dr. Bates' patients had exercised or recently drunk water it would have affected his results.

As we age, the eye loses length, so again if Bates was using older people in his studies of eye length, he may have misjudged the long term changes of aging as being representative of normal eye length changes.[lvii]

There is also the possibility that Dr. Bates was entirely correct, and the eye does change shape even in mature adults. It just is so slight that it has taken modern medicine until very recently to measure it. In countries like the U.K., discussions about changes in the length of the eye don't have the same level of tension. Researchers talk about "transient changes in the length of the eye" as part of the ciliary muscle's contraction. It makes sense that a ball of fluid is going to change shape slightly when it's squeezed in the middle. So Dr. Bates might have been right about the eyeball changing length during focusing after all.[lviii] He was just seeing change too subtle to be seen by his colleagues.

As recently as this morning I had a rather disconcerting reminder of the possibility that Bates was correct. While doing a single eye exercise (fading in and out on a page of small text which I call eye pushups), I distinctly heard the pop of my eye tendons as I moved my focus (not my eyes) rapidly in and out. The pop was similar to the sound we hear when flexing and turning our wrists and ankles. But I was using a single eye and moving straight in and out to exercise my inner ciliary muscles. No twisting or rotation should have been taking place. I repeated it several times until the sound faded, just as it does when I roll my ankles or wrists. According to modern optometry, nothing should have been moving besides my ciliary muscles within my eye. Yet I know what I heard and felt. Something on the outside of my eye was indeed shifting during my change in focus.

If we add all of the factors affecting Dr. Bates' research, the overall picture is not one of a fanatic. It is one of a researcher who has discovered a piece of the truth and refuses to let it go despite tremendous professional pressure. The effort may have cost him his health and perhaps even his sanity.

Dr. Bates was correct that the eye does not focus with the lens alone. He was correct that the eyes of many of his patients were changeable in length. Had Dr. Bates been more political about relaying his discoveries to his colleagues, he might be seen today as a founding member of modern optometry rather than a madman. His eye strain theory sounds exactly like "computer vision syndrome" back when it was "long hours in a sweatshop sewing in dim light syndrome."

While no one is apologizing to Bates for misjudging him, modern optometry is using what he discovered. The practice of Orthokeratology uses hard contact lenses to reshape the front of the eye overnight. The effect is a correction of the person's sight without any change in the lens of the eye. Using these lenses at night can slow the progression of nearsightedness among teenagers and aid a little in the current pandemic.[lix]

The greatest proof that the lens alone is not responsible for focusing our sight comes from the surgical practice of LASIK. [lx] In this surgery, the surgeon cuts into the surface of the eye (the cornea), leaving the lens untouched (but cutting the corneal nerves, leaving about 20% of patients with dry eyes).[lxi] Flattening the surface of the eye is enough to improve the vision significantly (about two lines on the eyechart)[lxii] and over a prolonged period (which gradually fades).[lxiii]

Bates' ideas about the eye shape change was right, he just made it too simplistic and ignored the lens. It was more than enough for his critics to disregard him. Rather than looking at the possible effectiveness of Bates' exercises, the optometric community has ignored eye exercise, claiming this one part of the body doesn't benefit.

A simple cost/benefit analysis reveals the flaw in this approach. Cost for the exercises? Nothing. Benefit of the exercises? Possible sight recovery. So why haven't Bates' style exercises gained wider acceptance?

7 Why Don't We Exercise the Eyes?

If there's no harm in exercising the eyes, why aren't more people doing it?

Remember, back in the 1920's the field of optometry wasn't what it is today. The people prescribing eyeglasses weren't really interested in people not needing eye glasses. They were busy building a profession, passing laws state by state so they wouldn't be jailed for practicing medicine without a license.[lxiv] So they would not have paid attention to a New York eye doctor named Bates promoting eye exercises even if he hadn't been a jerk about it.

But surely someone else must have thought about doing eye exercises since then? Well, there was this thing called the Great Depression, followed by World War II. No one was really looking at preventative eye care, they were busy trying to survive.

THE BALTIMORE MYOPIA CONTROL PROJECT

Near the end of the war, there was some interest in eye exercises. The American Optometrists' Association conducted a study of whether eye exercises prevented the need for glasses, the Baltimore Myopia Control Project. It was a joint venture, with ophthalmologists testing the patients before and after, and the optometrists doing the actual vision training. The optometrists were proving that they were part of the medical profession, and their rivals were setting themselves up as the judges of just how effective optometry was at helping the eyes. At the end, the judging ophthalmologists declared that eye exercises didn't help patients at all, while the optometrists said they did help. It was the ophthalmologists' medical opinion, not the upstart optometrists', that has carried on as "common knowledge" to the present day.

But "common knowledge" should probably have known better. A re-evaluation of the Baltimore Myopia Control Project data in 1991 completely changed the picture. Using modern methods of analysis, the researchers concluded the data supports the optometrists' old view. The true conclusion of the Baltimore Myopia Control Project is that eye exercises do help nearsighted people.[lxv]

What is striking about the 1940's study was that the very people who stood to lose the most business, the optometrists, found the most benefit for patients. Over a short period, patients doing exercises improved two lines of the Snellen eye chart. That's a significant and dramatic improvement, almost equivalent to getting LASIK surgery today.

But the ophthalmologists somehow concluded that the visual improvement was only one line of text on the eye chart (not significant). How could this be? The authors of the re-evaluation comment that bias might have been involved in the conclusions from the 1940's. The original study was not double-blind (the ophthalmologists knew who was getting the training and who was not). So they could make a decision about how well they thought the exercises worked.

What could possibly be gained by invalidating eye exercises? The Baltimore study mentions "widely publicized methods of visual training" as being the only reason for needing the study without mentioning Dr. Bates by name.[lxvi] But he was the reason they needed to show the standard method of eye care was the right one.

In a second eye exercises study in 1947, ophthalmologist Dr. Hildreth begins his discussion by declaring Bates' exercises have already been proven worthless. *"The fact that very few have been able to dispense with their glasses is sufficient evidence of the ineffectiveness of the method."* Then he goes on to say that they've improved on Bates' worthless exercises, but - guess what? - they don't help anyone either.[lxvii]

Forty years later, we know that these ophthalmologists doctored their data, burying Bates' exercises for all time with a pair of non-blinded studies that set out to prove him wrong. The medical authorities had spoken at a time when a white coat was always right.

As a result of these 1940s studies, later studies of the eyes began with the assumption that eye exercises could not permanently help nearsighted patients. In 1982, nearsighted patients used a computer program to improve their eyesight from 20/800 (nearly blind) to 20/25 (normal vision) without squinting. But the researchers did not conclude that the eye could be improved, because the lens of the eye had not altered. Instead, they concluded, *"The results are best explained by the formation of an artificial contact lens resulting from tear-film changes...a learned perceptual process may also be involved."*[lxviii]

Given the computer program's results, I would conclude

that the eyesight of the nearsighted patients was improved, clearly and dramatically. It doesn't matter whether we acknowledge that the front of the eye does change shape, which it clearly does from laboratory testing and the effectiveness of LASIK. We can make up "an artificial contact lens" made of tears if we want to. The point is that the patients could see better. Why didn't this study spark an industry of eye exercise programs? Yes, it was temporary, but a long term follow up study would have seen if the improvement could be permanent. Instead, the researcher makes it seem like the improvement of sight wasn't real. The patients instead responded to suggestion, somehow hypnotizing themselves into seeing better.

It's not the first time eye doctors have claimed that eye improvements were self-delusion. Even during his life, Dr. Bates was hounded for "hypnotizing" his patients, making them think they could see clearly when they could not. One prominent patient of Bates went around telling people how unethical Bates was for hypnotizing him after Bates cured him of his forty year need for glasses in fifteen minutes. After his improvement the patient went around asking other prominent eye doctors how this was possible, and was told it simply was not. Later the patient's eyesight returned to its previous nearsighted state. He came to believe that Bates must have used some trick. And perhaps Bates did. Today we know that hypnotism does not change the eye.[lxix] But it can change how well people think they see.[lxx] The process of relaxing the eye, regardless of how it is accomplished, seems to be beneficial. So Bates was changing how his patients thought about how they saw, and they saw better. Until other authorities told them it was impossible, their eyes tightened, and they saw worse again.

The biggest "proof" of the lack of benefit from eye exercises comes from China. In 1963, the Chinese authorities mandated five minutes of eye exercises every day for students. So for fifty years we have children trying to improve their eyes five minutes a day. Does it make any difference? Yes and no. Media articles will claim no effect from all these exercises.

"Despite these eye exercises, rates of myopia in urban China have soared to nearly 90%, according to recent studies. 'China has among the highest rates of myopia and it's the only country in the world that does eye exercises, so it's probably not working all that well,'"[lxxi]

But analysis of the exercises shows a benefit from doing the exercises correctly just once. Researchers looking at the way the exercises are done showed:

"many children thought it was boring to do eye exercises and preferred to use the time to study... 97% of school age children did not know the correct pressure to do (the) eye exercises"[lxxii]

If we did a study in the U.S. on eye exercises and 97% of the people did it wrong, we would not conclude that the exercises did not work. We would conclude that the people setting up the study didn't do a good job of teaching their subjects how to do what they need to do. So the Chinese eye exercises aren't evidence of anything other than kids can do things wrong and that U.S. experts have a bias toward declaring eye exercises useless.

At the same time, the Chinese have documented a significant decline in vision over that last twenty years. So pupils simply maintaining their vision with a few exercises without declining could be significant.[lxxiii]

For patients with one of the worst eye diseases, macular degeneration, giving them the ability to manage their own exercises improved their lives by *"reducing distress and disability, improving self-efficacy, and preventing depression"*[lxxiv] So even if the eye exercises do not cure the illness, the effects are very positive. The benefits on stress and mood also lasted at least six months after the end of the exercise trial.[lxxv]

For healthier people, more recent studies show that practicing seeing better results in - seeing better.[lxxvi] Healthy people who trained themselves to see changes in red or green light got better than a control group at seeing those changes and reacting.

But we all know that we can get better at our recognition and reaction times through repetition. We shouldn't need studies to prove that practicing a physical skill like sight improves function.

What about studies that still show no benefit to exercising the eyes? Even a study published in 2018 found that eye exercises have no value. But if you look at the study, the researcher is actually misrepresenting their own outcome. The small Indian study was done on eye exercises because 69% of Indians are now nearsighted. Neither Bates' eye exercises nor a Traditional Indian eye strengthening exercise were found to be helpful. In the summary, the authors concluded, *"non-pharmacological approaches such as eye exercises... are not significant on myopia."*

But fortunately the whole Indian study is free online, and a simple reading of the study showed that, while Traditional Indian eye exercises did not improve sight, Bates eye exercises showed a trend toward improvement over the few weeks of the study. In fact, that trend was significant. In the body of their article the same authors comment, *"it was seen that there was a slight reduction in the myopia by performing the eye exercises. Hence, it states that Bates eye exercise has significant effect over the refractive errors over the participants involved in this study."*[lxxvii] When is a significant result in eye improvement not a significant result when you summarize your research? When it involves the name of Dr. Bates. Almost a century after his death, the prejudice against him remains strong.

Other studies that aren't trying to disprove Dr. Bates show that even a ten minute round of aerobic exercise can improve the eye's function.[lxxviii] We've all experienced this as we "get into the game" and our reflexes adjust, including our vision.

When we look for improvement in our sight, we're looking for our eyes to feel better overall. Doing eye exercises can give relief to the majority of people practicing them, even if their objective results are only one line of improvement on the eye chart after three weeks.[lxxix]

Let's put that kind of "insignificant" improvement in the larger context of the ongoing pandemic of nearsightedness. For comparison, those three weeks of exercises gave about twice the benefit a year's worth of our best eye drug is expected to give nearsighted children. And those exercises can be used with a lot fewer side effects than the drug.[lxxx]

When we look at these studies and reflect on our own experiences with our eyes, it just doesn't make sense to disregard the benefits of practicing seeing better. Do we look for studies on whether practicing the piano helps? While we normally don't practice things like smelling or hearing, clearly both of these skills can be improved in professional wine tasters and concert-level musical performers. So sight is not unique among the senses. It, too, can be improved with practice.

8 Why Does The Eye Get Worse?

We might not know how to make eyes better in our society, but at least we know why they get worse, right?

Not really. The standard answer for the worsening of eyes seems to be a combination of genetics and bad luck. Eye researchers are looking constantly for more genetic markers. These new markers will tell unfortunate patients just how high their chances are going to be of getting retinal detachment or macular degeneration - just like their parents.

According to the genetic researchers, if these illnesses don't run in your family you have much less chance of getting them. But many of the people getting these diseases now don't have a family history.

Rather than throwing out the idea that genetics cause eye diseases, researchers now say the relationship between genetics and eye health is "complicated." They say that since 90% of human genes are needed to make the eye, genetics really are the cause of things like degeneration and increased eye pressure.[lxxxi]

To the extent that without our DNA we wouldn't be alive and being alive is necessary to have an eye disease, they are right. But genetics doesn't explain much of the eye disease that we're seeing today.

For people who have poor eyesight and do nothing, they

can't expect to keep even their genetically poor vision. Over time, almost half of those with nearsightedness will get worse.[lxxxii] It doesn't help if they carry extra weight, smoke, and have high blood pressure.[lxxxiii]

We know that adding stronger glasses doesn't seem to make a difference in the progress of eye disease. Having younger children switch to bifocals made no difference in their eyesight over three years. What did make a difference in how bad their eyes got?

"the rate of progression tended to be the most rapid for subjects who entered the study at an early age with a large amount of myopia, and tended to be the least rapid for subjects who entered the study at a later age with a small amount of myopia"[lxxxiv]

In other words, the worse you are and the younger you are, the worse your nearsightedness is going to get. But is this just genetic? Or is it a result of the adaption of the young person's eye to ever-increasing nearsightedness and early glasses by lengthening itself further?

If we remember the example of Singapore, it moved extremely rapidly from a pre-industrial to high-tech society in the course of several generations. At the same time they were moving from agriculture to high-tech, the eyes of Singaporean children went from almost no nearsightedness (myopia) to overwhelming nearsightedness. Since the population of Singapore is mostly Chinese, the genetics of the island did not change.

What changed was a dramatic lifestyle shift, emphasizing school work and computer use over working outdoors or in fields. Somehow at the time I lived there I thought that the Singaporean experience demonstrated "common sense." The resulting nearsightedness is what we'd expect from a sudden societal change which moves children from playing outside to studying inside. I thought this without ever applying that same idea to my own life or society. Only since beginning this book have I realized that my own sight loss coincided with moving to a new home, absent parents, and having cable television for the first time in my life. Living on a busy highway I couldn't go out and ride my bike anymore. So instead I stayed inside and memorized all the earliest MTV videos. I was using glasses by my second year of watching cable all afternoon.

DOES STAYING INSIDE AFFECT SIGHT?

But we don't need to rely on my "common sense." In the Singaporean example we have a control group for comparison. Children of the same Han Chinese ancestry who live in Australia were compared to similar children living in Singapore.

Australia has a very different overall work ethic (Sorry to insult any Aussie readers, but Australia didn't have to move as rapidly up the economic ladder). The result for Australian Han Chinese children is more leisure time spent outdoors. How much more? Almost four times as much time outdoors as similar children in Singapore.

The difference in nearsightedness in six-year-old genetically similar children is dramatic. Over a quarter of the six-year-old Singaporean children are nearsighted, compared to just 3% of six-year-old Australian children who share the same genetic background.[lxxxv] Researcher Ian Morgan summed it up this way, ***"If children get outside enough, it doesn't matter how much study they do. They don't become myopic,"***[lxxxvi]

It would be nice if he was right. Going outside helps, but it's not the entire solution. Once nearsightedness starts, going outside won't stop it.[lxxxvii]

If letting children outside helps nearsightedness, countries like Taiwan have been doing the opposite. A typical Taiwanese teenager goes from school directly to evening "cram school" to try and get ahead of her classmates. On the weekends the same teenager is in "cram school" rather than taking a break.[lxxxviii] Not surprisingly, the rate of nearsightedness has climbed from 4% of Taiwanese six-year-olds in 1986 to 20% in 2000. By the time they reach the age of twelve, 84% of Taiwanese children are nearsighted. One in four of these are very nearsighted, and complications from being very nearsighted have become the leading cause of blindness in Taiwan.[lxxxix]

Recognizing the crisis, in 2010 Taiwan instituted obligatory outside play. In other words, they brought back recess. The result has been a significant lowering in the incidence of nearsightedness. But outside play doesn't stop people who are nearsighted from getting more nearsighted. So being outside helps if you aren't nearsighted, but something else is involved once you start down the nearsighted path.[xc]

If near work and computer work can cause nearsightedness in humans, aren't there some animal studies that confirm this finding? It turns out there are, and other animal studies might show us how to make things better.

MAKING ANIMALS NEARSIGHTED

Let's start with chickens.[xci] If you want to make a chicken nearsighted, you put goggles on her so she can only see straightforward. (Momentary pause while we imagine hundreds of fuzzy chicks with tiny little aviator goggles.

Awww!) Since the little chick can only see straightforward (like staring at a blackboard all day), her eyes start to grow longer and she gets nearsighted.

Take that chicken with goggles outside, and nothing much happens. The chicken still can't see to the side, so she still gets nearsighted. But something about being outside does slow down the progression of the chick's nearsightedness.[xcii]

Researchers have explored different options about why that slowing occurs and found the "miracle substance" is violet light.[xciii] Not hard ultraviolet light, the kind that causes sunburns. Just violet light, the 1960's and 1990's "black light" bulb craze that makes white t-shirts glow. So if we had more near violet light exposure as young people, we might have less nearsightedness. Dance party, anyone? (I'm joking, get outside an hour a day if you can.)

Sunlight contains all the frequencies of light. Everything from heat on up is coming off the sun in huge quantities. Is it possible to get that same light exposure inside? How do our own indoor lights compare? Incandescent lights, those energy wasting hot bulbs, are actually OK at giving off the violet light our eyes need. But no school district watching pennies would use such wasteful incandescent bulbs. No, we use fluorescents.

How do fluorescents match up to the sun for producing violet light? Not so good.

But wait, we're not done. We're switching from funky flickering fluorescents to the new, cool LED lights. How are they when it comes to violet light production? Not so good either.[xciv] If you want an LED light to give off violet light, you need to buy one specifically for that purpose (they are inexpensive and evidently useful for odd things like hunting scorpions).

Now, we can't save the world's sight by starting a

campaign to return to incandescent bulbs. That's going to go over about as well as asking people with stoves to return to cooking fires. But we can put in one good, hot old bulb ourselves in our favorite reading nook. Sure, conserve energy in the rest of the house. But use a full-spectrum light when you really want to spend some hours looking at small print. Your eyes will thank you.

Anything from chickens to monkeys gets more nearsighted if you stick it in a small room with a blackboard or some image directly in front of it. It helps to put blinders on either side of the animal's head so it never uses its peripheral vision.

DOES STARING AHEAD LENGTHEN THE EYE?

So why would staring straight forward day after day lengthen the healthy, non-nearsighted eyeball? Just imagine holding any part of your body rigidly in one position for four, eight, or sixteen hours a day. The muscles and tissue around that body part would tighten, holding the part rigid.

Over time, the need to only look one direction would atrophy other muscles, leading to weakness in the other areas. As the body pushed itself to hold that position longer, the tension and atrophy would encourage the eye to hold and lengthen in its position. Remember, a longer eye requires less tension on the muscles at the front of the eye. The shorter the eye, the harder the muscles have to bunch up, and the longer the eye the more they can relax while you stare all day at something much closer than the horizon. Over a few decades, you should have some nice long "football" eyes.

MY JOURNEY TO WORSENING EYES

But we may not get the same result at different times in our lives. During my growth as a child and adolescent, my eyes remained the same size. But my head grew around my eyes. That head, and the bones of my head, formed around my eyes as they moved. As the bones grew they would surround the eyes as tightly as they could. If the eyes were facing forward all that time, of course the bones would support that presentation. That's why my eyes worsened as I was growing. But once my body stopped growing my prescription glasses haven't changed in decades. My head isn't growing anymore, and the underlying pressure on my eyes to lengthen isn't there.

So for a very long time my ability to see wasn't impacted as long as I wore glasses. This is true of grown people with even severe vision loss (twice as bad as mine). Once we stabilize, we can maintain. The worse our eyesight, the thinner the tissue at the back of our long football eyes, but still we're stable for long periods.[xcv]

Only as I've aged, my eyesight has been getting less and less able to function without those glasses. Now that I'm aware, I'm stunned that the blurry shapes of letters don't correct themselves as I walk forward toward the Snellen chart. It's like my eyes have learned to be lazy, to not even try to focus even as they approach closer to what they want to see.

I can see no better at three feet than I do at ten feet without my glasses (your results may vary, and that's why you need to check yourself). If I make an effort to see, I don't see any better even though I can feel my eyes straining. Forcing my eyes actually makes them worse, not better. My ability to focus, to tighten my eye muscles around my lens and to change the shape of my eye, has deteriorated to basically nothing over decades of depending on my glasses. All I do when I try is make things more blurry by straining.

It reminds me of patients I've had who I tell to relax their backs or necks and instead they tighten. Their muscles are no longer under their conscious control.

If instead of straining I relax my eyes, close them and picture darkness or a beautiful horizon, at least the top lines of the eye chart eventually come into focus. It took about three weeks of daily exposure before this level of relaxation was something I could do regularly.

For me to be able to see 20/200 when I'm normally 20/350 is pretty impressive. Yes, I'm sure my eye doctor would say I'm squinting, but I think I do a lot of squinting without any conscious physical effort. Going forward, if I'd followed the conventional path of ever-stronger eyeglasses I was going to do a lot of squinting, removing of my glasses and "eye tromboning." You know, that middle-aged dance move where we pull text forward and back to try and see it more clearly? Instead, with a little effort I've progressed to being able to read labels with my glasses on using even my weaker eye now.

It troubles me that I didn't even notice my loss of eye function until I could no longer get my atrophied football eyes to focus on reading. Just like any other body part, since I haven't used my ability to rapidly shift from far to near all day every day, I've lost it. Use it or lose it holds throughout the body, the eyes included.

But something more that my personal sloth may have affected my ability to see as I hit middle age. Instead, this loss of sight seems to be an accepted universal truth. A right of decrepitude, if you will. *'For almost everyone, the need for reading glasses is an inevitable part of the second half of life.'*[xcvi] One possible idea of why this happens is that the eye becomes less able to change shape as it ages. Instead of flexing (just as Dr. Bates said it did), the eye gets stiff.[xcvii]

But is this vision loss inevitable? Age, nearsightedness, and gender all affect vision, with adult men typically having eyes thicker at the back than adult women.[xcviii] While this holds across cultures from China to Europe,[xcix] adolescent men may have thinner eyes than adolescent women, leaving them more vulnerable to damage during those early years.[c] Nearsighted adolescent females show visual changes at different times of their menstrual cycle.[ci] For anyone medical, the variation in gender, age, and during our adolescence points to a possible connection between eyesight and hormonal levels. What makes me even more suspicious of hormonal effects is that the American Optometric Association says that these eyesight changes stop and stabilize again around the age of sixty.[cii] What else stabilizes at a lower level around that time for both men and women? Hormones.

We know that many eye diseases are related to hormonal levels,[ciii] and that women tend to have significantly more macular degeneration.[civ] Women are also more likely to be nearsighted (though being white is by far a greater risk factor in the U.S.).[cv] Nearsighted people, regardless of gender, have a lowered blood flow in the eye.[cvi] Nearsighted adolescents tend to have more hormones than their fellow students.[cvii] Hormonal levels drop as we age, and older patients with the wrong mix of hormones are more prone to arterial stiffness (and eye stiffness).[cviii]

Have large-scale studies been done on what lifestyle changes can help this degeneration? Of course not. After all, *"Presbyopia is the normal loss of near focusing ability that occurs with age."*[cix] You don't do studies to correct something that is inevitable. It would be like doing a study on reversing grey hair, which clearly never happens (except when it does[cx])
.

Interestingly, one of the newest treatments for our loss

of near vision as we age is inserting a little mini-reading glass lens into a person's non-dominant eye. The lens is only about six microns thick. How does this miracle insert work? By blocking out excess light and allowing your non-dominant eye to see things more clearly. "This creates a "pinhole camera effect," which expands the range of clear vision to bring near objects into sharper focus."[cxi] So I could literally have a pinhole implanted in my non-dominant eye to help me read text. Cost of the FDA approved implant? Around five thousand dollars. Cost of a piece of scrap paper and a pinhole? Priceless.

9 Eye Diseases

When we talk about eye health, there are so many different diagnoses that it can be easy to get lost. Many of these diagnoses are separate only because different doctors named them at different times in history.

If the question is whether a lot of research has been done on treating each of the diseases, the answer is yes and no. A great many different drugs and surgeries have been tried. But almost no one is dealing with prevention rather than treatment.

The underlying cause of many of the illnesses is a problem of blood and fluid flow within the eye. It's not so much an issue of the body having what it needs to repair the eye, but of that material getting where it needs to go.

How that slowed eye flow presents in the eye can change the diagnosis and how slow the flow is can profoundly impact how bad the illness will be. But we still don't even have a gold standard for monitoring blood flow in the eye (as of 2018).[cxii] So how are we to judge one drug study vs. another if they are using different measurement systems?

Rather than getting caught into the discussion of how

well we treat which diagnosis, I want to mention different diagnoses with a focus on the bigger picture of how to prevent the eye's deterioration and inflammation.

WEAR-AND-TEAR

Wear-and-tear in the eye can happen suddenly, through a traumatic event that causes injury to the eye directly or indirectly. It is often an acute medical situation, one that is urgent but which can be resolved fairly quickly and completely with intervention.

A common and serious wear-and-tear diagnosis is retinal detachment. It is a very scary diagnosis. The back of your eye is coming loose and an eye doctor will use a laser to "staple" it to the back of your eye again.

But there is a non-urgent version of the same problem, with bits of your eye coming loose called floaters. Maybe you've been looking at the sky and seen something floating across your vision. What you see is something floating inside your eye, casting shadows on the back of your eye the same way clouds cast shadows on the ground. If you inquire with your optometrist about your "floaters," they seem unconcerned. These things happen, you're told, nothing to be done about them. We ignore them medically and don't recommend any treatment.

Some of my floaters seem to be farther back in my eye, while others seem to be in the front portion of my eye. I notice most a floater that likes to stay in the center of my sight, like a small ball that bounces from word to word as I read. It's annoying, but I know if I allowed myself I could get to the point that I could ignore it. If we can ignore a gorilla in a basketball game or 99% of our incoming light, we can ignore a small shadow inside our eyes.

There are no studies on floaters and any treatment

except a surgery, or vitrectomy.[cxiii] If having someone suck out the floaters with a needle doesn't sound like much fun, it's time to name your floaters. Since normal eye fluid also contains enzymes that break down things like floaters,[cxiv] it would be lovely if someone did a study on floaters and enzyme intake for increased breakdown. But it is likely that the issue is not the enzymes, it's the flow of those enzymes into and out of the eye.

If you should, one day, have a lot of floaters and bright flashes in the corners of your vision, everything suddenly changes from a standard eye doctor's viewpoint. You now have retinal detachment, the sight-threatening tearing away of the lining of the back of your eye from the rest of your eye.

So what's the difference between having a few floaters and getting retinal detachment? How do we know how much to worry? Well, family genetics are supposed to raise our risk, and head trauma raises your risk a lot. If you get hit really hard, it can detach your retina. That makes sense. But what if you don't remember getting hit really hard? Or what if it was years ago? How do we keep our eyes from detaching on the inside? Nobody knows. We do know that having surgeries like cataract surgery can cause tears in the eye later on. So can having uncontrolled diabetes. But most people who have either surgery or diabetes never get retinal tears.

It's likely that the process of retinal detachment without trauma is a complex interaction of fluid dynamics within the eye. Fluid dynamics are the reason why airplane wings are able to help lift a metal plane because of their tilt in the fluid of the air. Since few eye doctors are also experts in fluid mechanics (including me) the underlying nature of the detachment is hard to understand.[cxv] But it is clear that slowing the flow using a technique called scleral buckling (making a fold in the outer surface of the eye) can be as effective as more intrusive surgical techniques that involve drainage.[cxvi]

What's also clear is that severe nearsightedness, having an eye that is really misshapen, can lead to retinal detachment. Of the young people now getting severe nearsightedness, researchers estimate between ten and twenty percent of them will be at risk of blindness from either wear-and-tear retinal detachment or inflammatory degeneration.[cxvii]

INFLAMMATION

Even more scary than retinal detachment is the gradual loss of your sight. The most common form of this is called macular degeneration, and it's the leading cause of blindness in the developed world. What causes macular degeneration, and what can we do to stop it? No one knows, but many drug companies can't wait to get their hands on a drug that might help. Currently there are trials of different drugs being injected directly into the eye to try and slow degeneration.

But long before we have macular degeneration we can have something happening to the pressure inside our eyes (glaucoma). The increase in pressure means that the exchange of fluid inside the eye has slowed down. If the pressure changes enough, it can deform the eye and cause a person to go blind. But even if it doesn't, glaucoma is a sign that degeneration is happening in the eye. It is the eye's version of high blood pressure, a sign of upcoming degeneration as the fluid in the eye is no longer flowing, no longer circulating nutrients and getting rid of wastes.

We currently treat glaucoma the same way we treat high blood pressure, by using drugs in the front of the eye to decrease it. While the pressure is controlled, we're ignoring the underlying causes of the increased pressure that may cause other degenerative changes in the eye.

I'm going to focus on this eye pressure increase in the front of the eye because the front of the eye is the last place in the eye to get nutrition. If your eye front is not doing well, chances are good that the rest of your eye may follow. The front of your eye is like a canary in a coal mine, the first place you'll see disease.

Why does the pressure inside the eyes change in the first place? After all our study, no one really knows.[cxviii] We're talking about the leading cause of irreversible blindness worldwide, and we're still not clear about why it happens?

Here's what we know. The fluid in the front of the eye is mostly water. Officially, it's created by cells near the front of the eye, and that fluid drips through to the front of the eye in a slow, steady stream. Many books and articles describe the flow as a "passive system." There is no pump, so the only issue is if the passive drainage gets blocked.

A CANAL?

It seems strange that none of the books I looked at talk about the canal that extends from the back of the eye to the lens of the eye. This canal, called the hyaloid, Cloquet's or Stillman's Canal (it's so unimportant they haven't yet bothered to settle on a single name) connects the artery from the back of the eye directly to the lens at the front. It's largely ignored by modern optometry because it's generally assumed to be a rare "artifact." But recent advances in computer-aided eye scans show that the canal continues to exist in the vast majority of healthy people.[cxix]

I'm not trying to rewrite the optometry textbooks here, I'm just saying that we've got a canal full of clear fluid coming directly from the back of the eye to the lens of the eye. Nobody thinks it does anything because we used to think it was dissolved and reabsorbed by the developing infant eye until very recently. If we were to imagine that this canal (with its three different names) actually brings fluid directly to the lens of the eye, then we might become suspicious that a breakdown or blockage of this canal might cause problems. It might even be possible to connect the breakdown of this canal in older people with the onset of cataracts in the lens. But as far as the official medical texts are concerned, the canal is still an "artifact" like the appendix or the gall bladder. Yes, we know now that the appendix stores good bacteria for the gut and the gall bladder stores material to help you process nutrients and fats, but that doesn't mean the canal does anything.

DRAINING

Whether it gets there by canal or is secreted by the cells, once the fluid gets into the front of the eye it goes around a couple of corners at the front of the eye (if it gets trapped that's a medical emergency).

The fluid empties out through a tiny hole in the front of the eye that connects to the veins on the surface of your eye. Yes, they call this tiny hole a canal (Schlemm's) but we know a tiny hole when we see it. The higher the pressure within the eye, the smaller the hole gets.[cxx] Yep, that's the problem. Your drain gets squished like a stomped-on garden hose when the pressure rises inside your eye, so it lets out even less fluid, increasing the pressure. That's the Catch-22 we call glaucoma.

The fluid we're talking about is lymph, the same stuff that gets ignored elsewhere in the body unless you've got a swollen lymph node in your neck or swollen feet because the lymph isn't returning up your legs. Lymph trickles between the tissues of your body in tiny little channels until it eventually returns to the heart.

The exit for the lymph in the eye isn't even a blood vessel, it's a tiny little canal path between cells. It needs to be fully open or you've got glaucoma. The place this fluid empties into is the veins on the surface of your eye. How fast does your eye canal path empty? We don't know. The veins on the front of your eye are so individualized, so unique, that they are used for identification purposes like a fingerprint.[cxxi] That's bad news if you're trying to do a study of a drug trying to increase this flow, because every patient is unique.

So what affects this flow in the front of your eye? Officially pretty much anything and nothing. High blood pressure can make it worse, but so can low blood pressure, particularly at night.[cxxii] Being a woman makes your chances of getting glaucoma more likely, so there has to be a hormonal piece to the flow. Being Asian increases your risk (part of the overall epidemic of nearsightedness). By 2020, ten million people worldwide will be blind from glaucoma.[cxxiii]

TREATMENT?

So can we do anything about the eye's flow? Officially, we give steroid drops to paralyze the eye's contraction and hopefully increase the flow out of the eye.

The flow changes throughout the day and is highest in the morning.[cxxiv] Since the flow is happening practically outside the body, changes in temperature on the surface of the eye can increase or decrease the flow.[cxxv] (Remember palming your eyes to increase blood flow?)

We're talking about an area the size of a dime that can be affected by temperature, so how many studies have we done on temperature and glaucoma? None. Researchers are just now discovering that sleeping with a pillow reduces glaucoma (one pillow helps, three don't help more).[cxxvi] That's the state of the research.

If we look at the physics of eye pressure, contracting the eye to see things nearby tightens the muscles and decreases the flow of fluid through the eye. Looking at the horizon and allowing the eyes to fully relax would increase the flow of fluid through your eye.[cxxvii]

Think of it like your hand. If you keep your hand tight in a fist, the palm of your hand will not get good blood flow. If you open your hand from a tight fist, you can see that your palm looks more yellow. Once you release your fist, your palm will rapidly get slightly pinker as the blood flow returns to your hand.

So if the eye is under greater tension when it is constantly used for close viewing, we'd expect an increase in glaucoma worldwide. We have an increase, but glaucoma strikes for a variety of reasons. One type of glaucoma is related to genetics and is highest in Africa (and the U.S. among African-Americans),[cxxviii] while a more aggressive type of glaucoma is more common in Asia. The biggest risk factor for glaucoma is not daytime stress, but very low blood pressure in the eye at night.[cxxix] Think of people with heart disease or diabetes who don't have good blood flow in their eyes at any point in their day. The loss of oxygen reaching the front of the eye at night kills off eye cells that then gum up the exit of fluid during the next day.[cxxx] In both sick and healthy patients, glaucoma is on the rise. By 2040, over a hundred million people will have glaucoma.[cxxxi]

We are currently treating glaucoma as part of a passive fluid system. But researchers monitoring the fluid coming out the front of the eye found that it does correspond to the pulsing of your heart, a little pulse like the end of a wave as it peters out on the sand.[cxxxii] So perhaps that "artifact" triple named canal coming up from the back of the eye might be pushing fluid forward into the front of the eye after all. If it is, then I wonder how many medical articles repeat the passive flow assumption without reexamining the eye for a connection between fluid from the back of the eye to the front. We might be missing the best chance we have to counteract eye degeneration by maximizing that canal flow. But I'm not an eye doctor, so why would they listen to me?

DRY EYES

If we're thinking about oxygen and the eye, we should at least mention dry eyes. The rate of dry eyes may be anywhere from seven to thirty-three percent of the population.[cxxxiii] It's worse if you're a woman, if you're older, if you smoke, and if you live in Asia. The biggest known risk factor for dry eyes is taking female hormones for birth control, which gives women five times the risk of having dry eyes.[cxxxiv]

You'd think we'd have a better handle on something as common as dry eyes, but the experts only came up with a complete definition of dry eyes in 2007. It hasn't been treated with respect as an illness.[cxxxv]

Remember, if your eyes are dry the front of your eye isn't breathing well. The lack of fluid means that it's hard for oxygen from the air to get into your eyes when they are open because the oxygen needs to dissolve in liquid before it can be absorbed by the eye surface cells. Even if you blink a lot, the eye needs constant moisture to get oxygen or nutrients.

The most common treatment we have for dry eyes is saline drops with different chemicals added, which we know isn't doing the job the tears are. It's keeping your eye from having to hold its breath all day, but it's like feeding a baby sugar water instead of mother's milk. Most experts recognize the deficiency, but have been unable to come up with a solution to deal with the body's lack of tears.

Strangely, we have a great solution if the tear duct is blocked rather than the tear gland. Usually tear ducts get blocked in infants. There is a surgery eye surgeons can do to unblock the duct but they rarely need to do it. Instead, eye doctors recommend parents massage the tear duct gently over time, which resolves the blockage 96% of the time. It can take months of daily gentle massaging to fully resolve the blockage.[cxxxvi]

What about massaging the tear glands and oil glands under the upper eyelid? Only recently have we had someone invent a machine to massage the upper eyelids to increase production from the tear and oil glands and help keep the eye moist. The result after twelve minutes was nine months of resolution for dry eyes after one session.[cxxxvii] But the inventors caution that the results are only preliminary.[cxxxviii]

If massaging the tear ducts takes months to fully resolve the issue, how many people with dry eyes have tried massaging their eyes a few times but given up because they didn't get any support from their eye doctors that it might help resolve their issue?

CATARACTS

Any overview of eye diseases should include cataracts, the cooking of the front of the lens. The current solution is surgery, making cataracts the most common reversible cause of blindness in the world.[cxxxix]

How cataracts form is an ongoing discussion, but we can

get some information from young patients with Ebola. As part of the disease, Ebola causes scarring in the retina of the eye. Most often it only scars the edges, so the patients don't lose their sight. But a few Ebola patients also get cataracts. In those patients, researchers found that the flow at the front of the eye was slow because the patients didn't produced enough fluid.[cxl] So too much fluid at the front of the eye can lead to glaucoma, and too little fluid can lead to cataracts. It may be possible to support the eye from the front using eye drops that absorb and alter the cataracts, but that research is still preliminary (we'll talk about those in the diet chapter).

By looking at wear-and-tear and inflammatory changes in the eye, I hope I've given a broader picture of the underlying reasons for many eye diseases. While you may personally have a rare eye illness, I'm hoping that knowing about inflammation and wear-and-tear will start you thinking about other treatment options you may not have yet considered .

10 Can The Eye Get Better?

Can your eyes improve? Regardless of the diagnosis? The short answer is yes.

I can say yes without knowing your particular situation because if you practice something, you will improve. If any of you were to reply that your eyes are deteriorating as we speak, my response would be the same. Your eyesight can still improve.

Why? Because, even though we think we see with our eyes, we don't. We see with our minds.[cxli] The amount of information you take in with your eye at this moment far exceeds what you think you see. Every moment you look at this screen, your eyes are taking in all the surrounding "background noise" of the room, your body, your glasses, and everything else that up to a second ago you weren't paying attention to and didn't "see" at all. We know this because when you do clever experiments you can get people to ignore things like women in gorilla suits walking through basketball games. The official name for this situation is "inattentional blindness."[cxlii]

But if we can have "inattentional blindness" then we can also have "intentional sight." That increased attention may not alter your eye, but it can fundamentally change how you see. Just as the mind can ignore a gorilla, it can also learn to pick out new visual cues and increase how well you use that information coming into your eyes.

How do you learn to see better? By training your eye to see the same way you would train your hand to type or your foot to shift from the gas to the brake pedal.

Yes, just like both typing and driving, initially it will require a great deal of conscious effort to see better. But as you retrain yourself over time your brain will change. The sorting and processing of the visual information you are receiving will alter. Eventually you will change your seeing habits and the new ways of seeing will seem effortless.

Over time you may be receiving less information from your eyes as they age, but you can be interpreting that information more efficiently. So the overall effect will be an improvement in your sight.

Techniques that improve brain reaction times to visual cues are already big business among professional athletes looking for improved game scores.[cxliii] If they can increase their jump shot percentage, we can increase how well we still recognize loved ones in old photographs. We're only asking for minor improvements, and studies show that even a few weeks of training can improve our reaction times just like athletes.[cxliv]

DO NOT TRY, DO.

To begin seeing better, we need to stop trying to see better. By trying I mean straining to see something without our glasses on. If you do nothing else, at least stop straining your eyes today and never start again.

Imagine trying to type with fists clenched or trying to drive with your knees locked. Of course you'd fail to improve. In my own experience, straining tends to make my vision worse, not better. Instead of seeing a blurry first line on the eye charts, all I see is a blur.

But our natural inclination is to tighten our eyes to try and see. We're going to force the eyes to obey us. It's about as useful as tightening our jaws to try and eat.

Instead of trying, allow your eyes to be where they are. Allow your eyes to see the way they want to. If it's a blur, that's OK. You need to be OK with the reality of where you are. Instead of fighting or denying, simply accept the current state of your eyes.

Being OK with the blur is the difference between the guy who takes up an exercise routine by walking vs. the guy who wants to do five hundred pushups the first day. You need to have a realistic understanding and acceptance of where you're starting from to have a reasonable chance at succeeding.

Once you're OK with where you are (not happy, just realistic) start exploring the blur. It's not all the same. Different angles are going to give you different results, changes in the blur. Looking up for me at far text is clearer than looking down. I notice changes in the clarity of the text as I move my head left and right. If I allow my eyes to just rest on a line of blurry text, I find that my eye starts trying different ways of focusing on it. The text will become clearer and then more blurry. Usually for me this blur happens as soon as I notice a bit of clarity and try to cling to it, to strain to make it permanent. I tighten my eyes, and of course return to the complete blur. The muscles of the eye are exploring, trying to make sense of my world without my constant lenses.

ATTITUDE

The attitude of acceptance and exploration are critical to the journey of improving your eyes. It's not a sprint, it's not even a marathon. Improving your eyes is a lifelong commitment to making the best use of what you have.

Before I started this book, I used to be angry with my eyes, frustrated at their lack of performance. Internally I'd yell at myself, ordering more from my tired, red eyes and misusing them to do more than they could handle. The only time I noticed my sight was when it was failing.

Now I appreciate what I can see, which is far more than I saw before. But I've also become aware of the global pandemic of eyesight loss, and I'm so thankful that I can see better than millions of other people. I'm also grateful that I live in a country where I've had lenses available to me, so that I haven't had to live my life blind. No, I don't approve of how we treat eyes as a whole, but I'm personally grateful to every eye doctor I've ever worked with for helping me see the best way they knew how. It's possible to both work toward improvement and also have an attitude of gratitude toward those who have tried to help you along the way.

DROP LENS WORSHIP

Starting the journey to better sight means changing your relationship with your lenses. No, you shouldn't dump them. But find out how much you really need them.

For me, putting on my eyeglasses in the morning was a sacred ritual. One of my greatest fears has always been losing my glasses. If I was looking over a cliff or out on a boat, my first priority was to secure my glasses. It was like a precious part of my own body could be lost. I remember my feeling of shock and betrayal when my "unbreakable" frames broke. It felt as if a body part had failed me.

Since working on this book, I've gone from wearing my glasses every waking moment to spending about an hour a day without them. Since I'm a packrat, I have all my older prescriptions that are slightly weaker and work fine for things like computer work (rigged up with attachable yellow sunglasses to reduce glare.) I've taken to wearing different lenses throughout the day, causing my wife much merriment as I wander about with my giant eighth-grade lenses. "Those look terrible!" she tells me. Yep, they do. Some fashion don'ts never become fashion do's.

Becoming creative with your lenses, really thinking about how you use them and how your eyes function without them, is going to make the biggest difference for you as long as you make it a long term habit.

TAKE THE LONG VIEW

The physical steps to practicing to improve your sight are not just moving the eyes around or using the newest eye chart exercise routine ("Now do jumping jacks while rolling your eyes!") These are the equivalent to starting a new diet.

Sure, you'll be really excited for the first couple of weeks. But over a month or two your excitement will fade. You'll forget to practice, then you'll feel guilty about not practicing. Then you'll yell at yourself, and practice a bit more for a few days. Eventually you'll see less and less results from more and more effort, and give up.

If that sounds familiar, it's because that familiar process is not limited to eyes. Anything that we try to do too fast and too hard with the body tends to fail. Every health program loves to trumpet its success stories, the few people who loved the program so much they adopted it as their permanent lifestyle. Health programs largely ignore all the people who fail. "They didn't follow the program long enough," is the answer always given. The proper response is that the program wasn't easy to follow long-term for most (almost all) people.

THE BARE MINIMUM

So let's start with the bare minimum you will need to do. **Get some way to measure your eyes current strength.** Heck, use this book text as a measure if you have nothing else handy (keep reading for instructions). Check your eyes ability to see, become aware of how your eyes function.

Pay attention to when your eyes feel better and worse. Do more of the things that make them feel better.

That's it.

Really? Yep. **Just keep doing that...for the rest of your life.**
Those are the magic words that every health program should be required to add at the end of their health claims. The "Just eat meat, no carbs" diets would become "just eat meat, no carbs, ...for the rest of your life." Suddenly they sound a lot less exciting and probably not really doable.

If your doctor said to you, "Take these five drugs, which cost all of your extra income...for the rest of your life." You might want some alternatives, because that program starts to sound a little expensive.

But "Be aware of your eyes, find out what feels better and do more of it...for the rest of your life," suddenly starts sounding a lot more powerful.

If you don't do anything else, paying more attention to what makes your eyes better and worse is going to make you more likely to do more of the things that make your eyes better. (Unless you want to go blind and like making your eyes feel worse, but then why would you be reading this book?)

NO MAGIC, JUST A CHANGE OF FOCUS

Notice, I didn't say your eyes would magically heal if you paid attention. I just said they are likely to at least slow in their deterioration simply because you're paying attention to what helps them feel better and doing more of that.

Years ago they studied factory workers on assembly lines. The researchers would do things like change the lighting, add lemon scents, play music, etc. Remarkably, every intervention helped, but only for a short time. They realized that it wasn't the nature of the intervention that mattered. It was simply because something had changed. When something changed, the workers paid more attention and did better jobs. If you pay attention to your eyes, they are going to appreciate it. The trick is to keep doing it...for the rest of your life.

ADD ACTIVE FOCUS

But you didn't pick up this book to read that simply paying attention will help your eyes. You want more. Good.

It's time to focus. The term we're looking for with your eyes is attentive focus. Using your eyes actively throughout the day. Noticing your surroundings. When you notice your surroundings, you move your eyes more. When they move more, the surface of your eye (where you focus) gets more oxygen. Think of attentive focus like adding a stream to the stagnant pond that is your current normal eye activity. Initially there won't be much change, but over a few weeks you'll see things start to gradually improve as the eye starts shifting into a new normal. What you should notice is spontaneously looking up from your work more, noticing the scenery, even seeing things in your room or house differently.

TAKE A LENS BREAK

Give you more to do? Fine. Take off your glasses more often. Learn what tasks and times you can easily do without them. Do you really need your glasses when you're sitting in the car in a parking lot, waiting for someone? Really? You need to see clearly while twiddling your thumbs? No, sitting and straining to see without your glasses isn't helpful. But relaxing your eyes, letting the world go by, is increasing their blood flow. Maybe even close your eyes while you wait, giving them a little rest while you twiddle your thumbs.

TAKE A SCREEN BREAK

Are you twiddling your thumbs, or is there a screen in front of your face? Want more to do to help your eyes? Put down your screen. Just put it down. Turn off all your notifications except for the people who depend on you for their very lives. Seriously, you can binge watch those cat videos once an hour as they stack up, waiting patiently. You don't need to spend your life with your eyes reacting to a dim screen, straining to see some click bait ad about something you're only vaguely interested in.

Straining to see the screen isn't great for your eyes. No, the screen isn't as powerful as the old televisions. But the safe distance is around a half meter, and extended closer exposure can increase the oxidation of your eye cells.[cxlv] If that isn't enough, trying to read in dim light is a recipe for worsening your eyes (my mom was right all those years ago). No, no one has done long term studies on eye strain causing long term problems. (Except the giant, global "study" on how it might be making our eyes worse.) We just know that an hour of screen use can cause dry eyes, burning sensations, and eye fatigue. If it was any other body part, we'd assume the constant pain wasn't great for that body part.[cxlvi]

Keep your phones, just binge on them for a few minutes every hour rather than constantly. Don't believe me? We have our new illness for the eyes, called Computer Vision Syndrome.[cxlvii] Doctors are already at work trying to find a cure (other than telling people to use their devices less than the current average of ten hours a day of screen time).[cxlviii]

EXERCISES

Now we start preparing for your eye exercises. So many exercises are just exploring what your eyes can do. Start with simple things like looking over your glasses at things. Learn to trace the frame of your glasses with your eyes whenever you remember, or at least every time you are stopped in traffic. If you wear contacts, try to see the edges of the contact, where it starts to get blurry. As you move your eye, does the contact move as well? How well is your contact sealed onto your eye? Does it change throughout the day? Don't worry, we'll get to lots more exercises in the next chapter, but first we need to talk about setting up for your exercise routine.

EXERCISE PREP

What should you do to prepare your eye for this new exercise routine? Should you go out and buy a special eye exercise suit covered with eye chart patterns and a matching green visor? Nothing new is required. If you eat horribly and don't sleep, that's where you're starting. If you already have a plan or program to help your eyes, there's no reason to change it - yet.

MEASURING YOUR PROGRESS

The first steps to exercising your eyes begin when you start measuring where your eye is now. If you have access to the internet, print out two eye charts, one for long distance and one for near vision. You can find the charts for free online at websites that want to refer you to nearby optometrists. The far vision (Snellen) charts are all standardized to the same size, but you'll usually find distance charts for ten feet away that are more useful (unless you have access to a twenty foot room). There is still no universal standard for the near vision (Jaeger) charts. New eye charts are in the works, because optometrists are realizing they don't have great, uniform tools to use and their standard chart is two centuries out of date (1863). So find one of each kind of chart that you like, because the ultimate goal is to create a repeatable test for yourself.

There's something to be said for familiarizing yourself with the process of deciphering letters without your glasses. It's not a skill most of us practice every day, so practicing it will make you better at it. You can make your own letter chart, using different sizes of the same font. Or even shell out the money for an actual Snellen chart, because that's what your optometrist will likely be testing you on. Working with letters will help you avoid anxiety tightening and straining when your optometrist asks you to read them.

Next, you need to find an area of your home or

apartment that is going to be your own measuring station. Putting up the eye charts in a way that you can see them in the same light, from the same distance, is important. After all, these charts are what optometrists will use to measure how well your eyes are doing.

The way you read these letters will be the final judge of how well your eyes are doing. They are considered an objective measurement of your eye health. Not practicing them is the equivalent of showing up at a track once a year after never running or even walking all year long. Your optometrist coach times your mile run and tells you how healthy you are. Then she tells you to not bother walking or running until this time next year. That's how we measure our eyes.

It makes complete sense that you should have the same ability to measure your eye performance at home.

MY SET UP

The home long distance eye chart is usually at ten feet, and I chose a linoleum line in my kitchen floor as the ten-foot mark. It's actually ten feet and four inches, but what is important is that it's an easily visible landmark for me. Using something like a piece of tape is another alternative.

The goal isn't perfection, it's finding a personal standard of measurement. Think of measuring your eyes yourself as being similar to seeing if you still fit into your favorite pants. Sure, we could use all sorts of ways to measure your weight or body size, but you know how your pants are supposed to fit. That's the kind of familiarity with your own vision that you want to have over time.

For me, the linoleum line has become familiar, though I now only measure myself officially once a week (it was daily for quite a while). I've also put up both the "tumbling E" distance chart as well as a letter eye chart. Of the two, I like working with the tumbling E better, but that's likely because it's more familiar since it's been up longer.

For the near vision chart, it's usually measured at fourteen inches from your eyes. I put both of my charts on the inside of kitchen cabinets, because I measured the distance from my counter to the cabinet as fourteen inches. I like being able to close my cabinets if I have guests and don't want to explain my sudden fixation with eyesight. But again, a piece of tape on the floor fourteen inches from the wall would work as well.

Once you have your charts, the other thing you need is a place to write down your results. I use a notebook and a pen. Check your left eye by itself, and your right eye by itself. Do it for distance and then for near vision. I put down the time of day as well, because I have found background sunlight matters a great deal (as well as how many hours I've spent looking at a computer screen). Other observations can go in the notebook, like whether you exercised, if you had any allergies, or if your eyes feel more tired than usual. All of these can affect your sight, but you don't know how much until you test yourself.

OBSERVATIONS ON PROGRESS CHARTING

From my own experimentation, I can say that light levels make an enormous difference in how well I see. Using dawn light and then turning on the overhead fluorescent light (I know, not optimal) improved my ability to see. In the dawn light, my right eye was hovering around the near vision chart number eight (middle to poor near vision). When I added the fluorescent light, my right eye suddenly realized it could see. It shifted from number eight to number three.

With effort (which means giving the eye a chance to adjust, breathing, and letting the eye take time to refocus) I was able to make out number one (perfect near vision) in my right eye. The difference was more light and giving myself time to adapt, two things I've never thought to ask for when sitting in my optometrist's office.

Before my current "eye kick" I remember trying to see the near vision letter chart in my optometrist's office. The place must double as the bat cave when he's not seeing patients. Even if I had perfect vision my eyes would be straining to see in that little light.

So number eight on the near eye chart would be my official sight if I relied on my first, dim-lighted, sight measurement. It's comparable to what I would be able to see in my doctor's office. None of us should get stronger glasses because our optometrist hasn't replaced his office bulbs or forgets to turn on the overhead light before asking us to read tiny text. Truthfully, I suspect my optometrist has been trying to get me to try bifocals for several years now. I'm not saying he did anything unethical. He just didn't make my text reading easier for me by forgetting to switch on a brighter light.

I've also found dramatic shifts in my ability to read text during different times of the day. It also matters a great deal whether I've been working in bright or dim light all day. So the time of day of my optometrist appointment could be making a difference in my prescriptions. Since I typically try to "batch" my eye appointments with my children, I have been seeing my eye doctor late in the day. Remember that a too-strong prescription will force my eyes to accommodate. By waiting until late in the day, I'm getting the strongest glasses because my eyes are at their weakest. During the rest of the day, I'm over-accommodating and likely gradually worsening my prescription To his credit, my optometrist has recommended a separate prescription for computer work, one that isn't as strong. I said no because I figured he was just trying to sell me unnecessary glasses. But now that I understand my eyes better I'm likely to take him up on his offer.

IS THERE ANY PROGRESS?

Even in the short time I've been measuring, I can say that my vision has improved. As the economics professors would say, that which is measured can be managed, and that which is managed tends to improve.

The most important thing to realize is that your eye progress is the same as the progress with any other body part. Slow-and-steady wins. If I get up well rested, my eyes see better. My right eye can read near vision well, and my left eye can make out the long distance top letters. But if I've spent the day straining my eyes, the eye charts are a blur. We wouldn't expect the same performance from our legs if we've just run a marathon. The eyes are the same, you've got to know how they respond to the day's activities.

MORE TOOLS

I already asked you to get a Snellen chart and a near vision chart. You can also try the Hart charts, which are like dumbbells for your eyes, forcing you to focus far and near as you alternate reading the large print with the small print (these are more useful for people with better vision). What I've noticed in myself with a little use (three minutes or less) of the Hart charts is that my ability to "see" the letter E on the charts is better than the other letters. But

I've been practicing trying to see the E on the long distance "tumbling E" chart for several weeks. So already my brain has learned to "see" the E better than other letters when I'm doing the Hart chart exercises.

There's also a Tibetan eye chart that has never inspired me, but have fun with your nose pressed to the wall at its center as you peer around looking at the edges of the design.

I wouldn't invest in an online program for eye improvement until you've gotten the basics down. If we just walk through the idea of adding more screen time to improve your eyes, I hope you can see that it's a double-edged sword. The last thing I need is for someone with eye problems straining away at what is basically a boring computer game for hours in an effort to improve his or her sight.

EYE ATHLETES

Not satisfied by my gentle exercises in the next Moving Your Eyes chapter? So you <u>really</u> want to exercise your eyes? Time to think like a Kathakali dancer.[cxlix] Never heard of these eye gymnasts? The Kathakali dance in southern India goes on for a full day at a time, and the dancers never speak so eye movements are a big part of how they express emotion. A young dancer may practice eye strengthening by sitting up all night with the full moon and circle his eyes around the moon, alternating directions, the whole night long. So if you feel the need for some serious eye movement, spend a little time learning some basic Kathakali dance eye movements.[cl] I expect that will be enough exercise for even the most hardcore of you (the ultramarathon eye runners out there).

11 Moving Your Eyes

The reality is that we cannot prove doing eye exercises will save your eyes or even improve your eyes. We can't even claim that eye exercises will slow the progress of any eye illness.

MOVE YOUR BODY

But we can say that moving your body does make a difference in almost every eye study. Moving your body means moving your blood. Moving your blood means changing the pressure and motion of the fluid within your eye. Doing that every day slows the progression of disease and helps your eyes repair.

The opposite is clearly true. People with eye issues from too much blood sugar who sit around all day are at a much greater risk of losing their sight.[cli] Exercise can almost double the amount of blood that reaches the eye.[clii] So if you don't have a body exercise routine, that's the first step to any eye exercise routine. What should you do? I researched this extensively for another book (The Colon Cancer Diet) and the short answer is an hour of walking a day. For eye specific help, put your glasses in your pocket during the walk if you can do so safely. Beyond the walking, which maximizes the body's repair cycle, we don't have good studies on whether aerobics, Pilates, yoga, or anything else can help your eyes more.

EXERCISE: RELAXATION

In a couple of seconds, I want you to close your eyes and leave them closed for a long ten count. While they're closed, I want you to try and relax the muscles around your eyes. Go ahead.

I always have trouble with this exercise. Some of my muscles will relax, but others tighten up. One eye will get more relaxed than the other, and for the life of me I can't get the tighter eye to fully relax. In a Japanese study trying to lessen the effects of screen time, the researchers found that half of their Asian female subjects were unable to relax their eyes fully even after two minutes of computer training helping them. [cliii]

EXERCISE: TENSION

Now let's do a second exercise. In a few seconds I want you to close your eyes and tighten the muscles around your eyes. As long as it's not painful, go ahead and tighten them as much as you can. Tighten them for a count of three and then let them relax for a count of seven.

I find this exercise much easier. The increased tension brings on some interesting bright lights behind my eyelids, and when I release my eyes feel more relaxed overall. But the point of the exercises is not to find out which is easier, it's to take a few moments to nourish your eye. Both relaxation and muscular contraction are moving blood and fluid around in your eyes.

MORE IS NOT BETTER

While eye exercises may be helpful, it may not help to beat up on your eyes all day long. A massive muscular eye routine may not generate the necessary improvements in the eye.

What researchers have found is that dopamine release within the eye helps it repair and improve.[cliv] Dopamine is that same substance that is released by gambling or video gaming. It is addictive to the brain because it makes the brain feel better. We're not sure how to increase dopamine release inside the eye, and injecting people with dopamine just increases their eye pressures.[clv] In animal studies too little dopamine and too much dopamine can be a problem.[clvi] But increasing dopamine likely doesn't involve forcing the eye around. The opposite, like looking in a relaxed way at beautiful images, seems likely to be of more benefit for dopamine release. In the same way, playing outside and enjoying yourself may have far more benefit than thirty minutes of daily eye calisthenics. The attitude you have about the eye movement may be more important than the movement itself and that benefit may literally be a biochemical change in the eye.

Dopamine is also created from tyrosine, which is also essential for generating thyroid hormone. In Asian countries there still isn't monitoring of thyroid illness. When they do check thyroid levels they may use a wider range of normal, so it's hard to know if thyroid deficiency plays any part in any lack of dopamine and increased nearsightedness.[clvii] But it certainly makes sense to check someone with severe nearsightedness for low thyroid.

If you have enough dopamine in your eyes, it still needs to be released by light exposure. So doing any kind of eye exercises in the dark isn't going to slow the growth of your eye toward being more nearsighted.

How much light is needed for the eyes? In chickens, the nearsightedness slowed as the chicks were exposed to stronger and stronger light up to ten thousand lux.[clviii] A lux is a unit of brightness, and many lights for Seasonal Affective Disorder use that same amount of brightness (ten thousand) for the prevention of winter depression. Think of a photographer's professional lights, the ones that are so bright they don't shine them directly on you. Those are the right level of brightness. Having experimented with a 20,000 lux light, it's still no match for sunlight in brightness or ease of sight, but it's as bright as indirect daylight. The sun, if you're wondering, starts about thirty-five thousand lux and moves up to one hundred and twenty-five thousand lux. We just don't have a lamp that mimics the sun.

It's also not going to be helpful to do more anaerobic exercise, the kind that doesn't use oxygen to generate muscle response (think weight lifting). Starving the body for air while doing the new Paleo upside down kettle bell weight routine isn't likely to do as much for your eyes as taking a long walk for about an hour a day. Your eyes need oxygen, and the muscles of your eye do crunches all day long already. What they need is more oxygen and a little distance viewing so they can relax and enjoy it. So a combination of eye exercises with a breathing routine may be helpful. Research participants who did both eye exercises and breathing as part of a yoga routine improved their eye sight significantly.[clix]

But, frustratingly, you may not see any immediate

improvement in your eyesight even if you're doing things right. Realize that our background reality is progressively worsening vision as we age.[clx] So even staying at the same level of eyesight over time can be a bit of a victory.[clxi] Recognize that, while objective eyesight may not be improving, you can speed up your reaction times to stimuli in your environment. Doing so can be lifesaving, as patients with eye illness can have delayed responses to dangerous hazards.[clxii]

HOW GOOD CAN IT GET?

How much improvement can we truly expect from eye exercises alone? After all, whether from genetics or from misuse, the eye can be truly misshapen. What is the average expected improvement of the eye from just maximizing the muscles without changing the shape of the eye? We don't know. In fact, the official take on exercises is that none of them work, even for children. Oh, except when it comes to making the eyes track together (lazy eye treatments).[clxiii] Those work. Also the recovery from cataract surgery, where your eye has to relearn how to see with a plastic lens. Exercises can help that recovery. But those are the only exercises that are recognized to work. So we don't have good measurements of what the nearsighted or farsighted eye could do by maximizing its muscular contraction.

But we can estimate, based on how well the eye bends light at rest vs. how well it can bend light when it's under maximum muscle tension. The combination of our eye lens and the front of the eye gives an average person a light bending power of about fifty (diopters) at rest. When focusing light under maximum muscle tension, the average eye gets a light bending power of about fifty-four. So "the muscles of the eye must provide an accommodation range of 4"[clxiv] OK, what does that mean in English?

For those of us with eyeglass prescriptions, our prescriptions are written to give the light bending power (diopters) of our eyeglass lenses. My current prescription is - 3.50 in one eye. That's three and a half, just shy of the normal maximum light bending power of the average eye, with the negative sign being nearsighted. If I was farsighted, it would be a plus sign.

If you don't have a prescription, normal vision is 20/20 and requires a prescription lens with the light bending power of zero (no lens). The numbers 20/20 stand for seeing at twenty feet what you should see at twenty feet. Basically, you can read the Snellen eye chart like you should.

Add roughly half a light bending power for every ten feet of nearsightedness if a person is close to normal.[clxv] A person with 20/40 vision would need a lens with the light bending power of -1.00. They can see at twenty feet what a normal person can see at forty feet. Adding a thin lens will correct their vision so they can see at twenty feet what they should.

As the lenses get thicker (the "coke bottle bottom glasses" look) the ability of the lens to bend light goes up quickly. A person with a lens with the light bending power of -2.00 can see without glasses at 20 feet what a normal person could see at 150 feet. A person with -3.00 lens can see at 20 feet what a normal person could see at 300 feet. Since I'm -3.50, I can see roughly at twenty feet what a normal person would see at three hundred and fifty to four hundred feet away. Yep, most of the world is a blur, or what I like to think of as a Monet or other Impressionistic painting. All I can see are the colors.

But, most importantly, despite living in Blurville I'm still within the range of what my eye muscles should be able to accommodate. In other words, even my poor eyesight (a blurry large "E" if I'm lucky on a regular eye test without glasses) should be entirely correctable by my eye muscles if I could just use them properly.

But maybe I'm too old? When children have lazy eyes, wearing an eye patch on the other eye is very effective before they are seven years old. Afterward, it's supposed to be permanent.[clxvi] But that assumption is based more on dogma than data. More recent studies on lazy eye have shown substantial vision recovery is possible in both adult animals and adult humans.[clxvii]

So how do we begin to maximize our eye muscles? When we think of moving the eyes, we think of the eyes rolling in their sockets. But there are four types of eye movement.

QUICK JERKS

The first type of eye movement is quick and jerky. Think of the eye under the eyelid during sleep. It's moving quickly back and forth. These motions are called saccades, and are largely involuntary. We hear something, see motion, and our eye locks on the moving object. The motion is run by the base of the brain. But it can also be done voluntarily, darting the eye from one focus to another. The Hart eye charts use this, as does much of the ball catching done in athletics. If you want to practice saccades, using the different points of the eye clock and focusing on the most peripheral points (the farthest your eye can stretch) will maximize this exercise. It's hard to do without moving the head, which happens automatically as we track the object we want to focus on.

SMOOTH TRACKING

Smooth pursuit movements are the opposite of saccades. The eye tracks the object to keep it in focus. If you've ever followed a fly or an airplane in the sky you've used smooth tracking. It's almost entirely voluntary. But only skilled people can make a smooth tracking motion with their eyes when they lack something to track. Practicing smooth tracking of objects at various distances would be the best way to get this skill up to speed. Try to get to the point where you no longer need an object. When I try this, I find that I'm imagining following an object, but that my eye jumps (saccades) several times during the motion.

CONVERGENCE

While we rarely think of it, the third kind of eye movement is looking at our noses. It's vergence movements, which really means convergence. Glasses make this kind of exercise unnecessary, so it is the number one way to start exercising your eyes. It's useful to do this with a single eye, feeling what happens when you move the focal point closer and farther away. Then try lining up the focal point of both eyes together at different distances so that you get a single image. Trying this simply by keeping your eyes on your finger as you touch your nose. If you pay attention to the background, it shifts as your eyes literally turn toward each other and you get overlapping images. But you can also allow vergence to lapse at any distance and then bring it back into focus. The best way to practice this might be 3D "magic" stereograms, where you allow your vergence to lapse just a little and use the two eyes to create a 3D image from the differences between them.

HEAD COORDINATION

The last eye movement can't really be done from an armchair. It is the vestibulo-ocular movement the eyes go through to keep an object in focus even though the body is moving. Watch this page and turn your head from side to side. Now tilt your head and swing it back and forth while trying to read. Sorry, but this is the part of the movement where you get up and dance, at least do a twist in your chair. Each body motion forces automatic adjustment in your neck, head, and eyes to keep the text in focus. It's this coordination that takes a long time for babies to master, and that we lose if we spend a long time on a ship and then return to land. The automatic nervous system coordinates the inner ear (the vestibule) with the eye (ocular) and compensates for sudden motion by making an automatic compensation. Bounce around for a minute and marvel at how incredible your system is that you can read words while bouncing up and down or rocking from side to side.

The same system that keeps your eyes level can also save your neck if you trip. It literally sets up an automatic reflex to pull your head up and out of the way while telling you to put your hands out and to bend your legs. All of this while your mind is still thinking, "Oh, oopsies." Thank goodness for our automatic systems.[clxviii]

PUTTING THE EXERCISES TOGETHER

Any number of different exercises can maximize your four types of eye motions. Rather than assume one set of exercises will meet all needs, experimentation is the key. Try each of the different types of motion. If they all feel natural and easy to you, wonderful. If not, notice the areas where you are uncomfortable. Those are the first places I would focus, practicing those motions until they feel natural. Think of it like relearning to walk after a surgery.

You need to be patient but consistent about making sure that your weak eye or weak area of motion gets stronger.

Once you can easily do all the motions, it's time to combine them. A quick look at the Bates Method of eye exercises shows that he was combining several different eye motions, but focused first on relaxation. It's important to make sure your eyes are relaxed throughout. If you begin to strain, you're making things worse.

There are many, many exercises online that both use and expand on Bates' original exercises of palming (covering the eyes with the palms), central fixation (gazing in a relaxed an non-focused way), swinging (smooth tracking of a stick or pencil from side to side), sunning (letting the sun play on your closed eyelids, which leads to relaxation), and shifting (gazing from near to far to near). All of these are basic, easily done, and effective without any further exercises being necessary…if you do them for the rest of your life. For full details, Bates' book is available online for free, and chapter fifteen has multiple shifting exercises.

MY CHANGING ROUTINE

Let me add some of the many exercises I have created for myself. In my experimentation I have already tried dozens, if not hundreds of variations. Many of the things I thought should work haven't, while others have worked well.

These are the ones that I have found most useful for me. In the process of finding what helps me I may have done and discarded exercises that might benefit someone with a different set of circumstances. One day we may have a specific set of exercises available for each type of visual issue, just as we do for different muscular issues. But until that time, let me give you what I have with the hopes that it may spark your own ideas for yourself.

MAKE FRIENDS WITH YOUR EYE CLOCK

Before bed or in the morning, stretch your eyes. If you don't feel like Kathakali level stretching, remember there is a clock technique for stretching based on Feldenkreis' work.[clxix] Basically you look up at twelve o'clock, over to your right at one, then two, three, and so on until you get back up to twelve.

I usually do this once each direction when I remember, and often find that I've got one or two painful directions that makes me take a few seconds to stretch that eye muscle until it eases off and I can go on. Just like your neck or shoulders, your eyes' muscles can get stiff.

Of particular interest in this clock stretch are the two o'clock position on the right eye (ten o'clock on the left) which is stretching one of the two oblique external eye muscles fully. The other oblique eye muscle is fully stretched when your eyes are at seven in the right eye (5 on the left), which means you'd be crossing your eyes to stare at your nose if you did them both together.

Unless you're terrified of being attacked by pigeons and are always glancing up and out, chances are you rarely use the ten and two in your peripheral vision. And unless you have a job threading needles, chances are good you don't look at your nose often with both eyes.

I bring these two muscles up because Dr. Bates believed these two muscles alone were responsible for focusing the front of the eye. He did experiments where paralyzing these muscles in animals reduced or eliminated the ability to focus the eye, and I have not found other animal experiments disproving these claims. Downside of stretching these muscles? None. You can spot pigeon attacks or food on your nose more easily. Upside? A possible connection between these muscles and your ability to see into the distance better.

We often assume that our eyes live in a vacuum when they are very connected to everything that is happening in the body, especially the neck and shoulders. If your body is crooked, the eyes will try to get the neck to twist so that they are even. We were set up this way so that we could see around ourselves even if injured. So stretching your shoulders and neck has the effect of increasing blood flow to the eyes while allowing their "support structure" to realign. Yes, this holds true all the way down the body. If your hips are off, then your neck is off and your eyes may be straining to keep things even.

EYE CLOCK (ONE MINUTE)

The eye clock is my basic stretch, one that resolved the optic migraines I got when I was in college. I call them migraines because my eyes hurt so badly I had to just go to bed. On the second or third one, I began slowly to stretch the muscles of my eyes. I would start up at twelve o'clock, then shift slightly to the right at one o'clock. Once that had eased, I moved a little more right to two o'clock, looking as hard as I was able in that direction until the tension and pain eased. Slowly working my way around the clock numbers released all the different combinations of my eye muscles and relieved my pain. Every night if I remember I will do the stretch, which takes about a minute unless I find an area of tension. In that case, it takes as long as the tension lasts to relieve it. I started this stretch after doing the home audiotape series of Moshe Feldenkrais, who uses the clock release for all parts of the body.

PARANOID EAGLE

Stare up and out at the edges of your outer eyebrows. Watch for pigeon or other bird attacks, but mostly stretch your internal oblique muscle.

THREAD THE NEEDLE

Stare at the end of your nose. See if you can see the tip while stretching the superior oblique eye muscle.

<u>A MINUTE FOR YOUR EYES</u>

JERKY CLOCK (5 SECONDS)

I practice glancing quickly at the twelve points of the clock in opposition (1-7, 2-8, etc.). This takes a few seconds but refreshes the eye.

SMOOTH CLOCK (10 SECONDS)

I practice tracking slowly between the twelve points in opposition, then roll my eyes both ways around the dial.

DRUNK GUY (20 SECONDS)

I touch my finger to my nose, tracking tightly with both eyes so my eyes cross. Then I do the same action with first one eye closed and then the other.

BOBBLEHEAD (20 SECONDS)

Keeping your eyes on a fixed location, shift your head around like it was attached on a string or you were a bobblehead doll.

All of those should be generally helpful for most eye issues. The following are what work for me because of my nearsightedness and the unevenness of my vision. I have a dominant left eye that also sees worse than my right eye. If you have the opposite problem, then swapping eyes would make more sense.

FASHION GLASSES (VARIABLE)

I have a collection of old eyeglasses (gathered together for donation, but kept for sentimental reasons). Trying on my different glasses, I am provided with a variety of visual experiences. Variation is a wonderful thing for the eye, and several of these eyeglasses are now part of my exercise routine.

PIRATE (VARIABLE)

Closing my dominant right eye, I read with my left eye. The result is often a straining to see with my right, and a feeling of frustration, of blindness, that I don't experience without my glasses. So I must close my right and periodically consciously relax it as I read with my left.

PIRATE PATCH (VARIABLE)

Instead of closing my better right eye, I have a child's cloth pirate patch that I put over the right. The result is better for the right, since holding the right eye shut tends to strain it. But most of us don't walk around with an eyepatch handy, so outside the home I just close my right eye.

FADE OUT (30 SECONDS) OR EYE PUSHUPS

Start with your nose against the page and move out. I have found that coming into a comfortable viewing distance results in constant strain right up to the point of proper focus. Instead, starting with the text up against my nose and gradually shifting outward allows me much greater control. By having the text too close to see, I have forced my eye into maximum focus. Gradually moving the text away allows me to hold that focus rather than straining to attain it from a distance. Just doing this exercise alone will improve your eyes.

RELEASE THE OPPOSITE EYE (10 SECONDS)

It's an unfortunate reality that the eyes want to work together. That means that the better eye will try to help the worse one see better. But it also means that the better eye may join the worse one if the worse eye is also the dominant eye. My right eye sees better if it doesn't have to deal with the left eye. But the left eye can also see better if it isn't trying to deal with the right. The two don't track together as well as they should. I think that the combination of poor tracking and the slightly drier left eye have contributed to it being worse than the right. But as I try to correct the left, I need to constantly release the tension in the non-seeing right eye as it struggles to "help" the left.

STOP TRYING TO SEE THINGS TOGETHER

One of the most interesting things I've learned to do is to allow my gaze to relax. Instead of staying steady, my eyes tend to cross. The tension to turn inward is greater than the tension to turn out, so they pull together. As they do that, both eyes are better able to focus. It's as if my eyes can do one of two things, either track together or focus, but not both. Releasing my eyes, letting them relax, and then working on allowing them to focus, rather than forcing them to focus, is helpful.

ALLOW YOURSELF TO BE BLIND

Every time I try to see, I get worse. Let me make that perfectly clear. I have noticed that my eyesight is extremely variable. In the morning I can see better than if I'm tired at night. If I work on the computer my eyes are worse than if I go out for a walk. But my eyes are consistently worse when I try to see.

I don't want this to be the case. It's very frustrating to have a glimmer of clearer vision that slips away. I'll notice a few letters clearing up. A line on my near or far vision charts seems tantalizingly close. But as soon as I lock on to that view, the moment I tighten, I lose it all.

One of my patients challenged me after reading an earlier rough draft of this book to test myself. If I think a child can change the back of her eyes in a few hours, can I change my vision in a few hours? The answer after several hours of trying is yes. Disturbingly so. After several hours in sunlight I was able to made out numbers at eight feet clearly with either eye. But not together. Both eyes together, focused on the same numbers, were blurry. When I relaxed my gaze, allowed my eyes to cross rather than holding them in alignment, I could briefly read the numbers clearly with either eye. But as soon as I grasped onto that clarity, strained to hold it, it was gone. I know what is happening is that my individual eyes are able to experimentally find an area of clear viewing on the bumpy, uneven back of my eye. And they can do it as long as they don't have to coordinate those points together.

The only way I found these points at all was by allowing things to be a blur. My eyes spent a great deal of time not seeing much of anything. But over time my eyes learned to accommodate, to reinterpret the signals they were getting.

NINETY SECONDS TO SIGHT

One of the things I did prior to being able to see numbers clearly at eight feet was to engage what I know about the involuntary contraction of muscles. Specifically, I know that involuntary contraction tends to ease if the opposite muscles are engaged. The time needed to ease isn't set, but a good rule of thumb is that it takes about a minute and a half of opposite contraction for the first set of muscles to release.

My relaxed eyes tend to drift inward and downward. Based on my basic understanding of the eye muscles, this corresponds to the pull of the superior oblique eye muscle. You don't need to know the name, but I mention it because Dr. Bates did animal experiments showing that the two oblique eye muscles, superior and inferior, were involved in focusing the eye. I'm not saying he's right, I'm just noting that one of my obliques seems to be a little overtight. So I engaged the opposite motion, looking upward and outward for ninety seconds (the Paranoid Eagle stretch above). Only after releasing and allowing my eyes to relax did I notice the momentary clarity of the numbers. Remember, I'd been relaxing my eyes for several hours at this point without successfully improving my vision without squinting.

WHY DO YOU NEED TO BE FULLY OPEN?

Every eye experiment notes whether or not the subjects were squinting. The reason is simple. We know that opening or closing the lids affects your sight. Specifically, opening and closing your lids changes the amount of light the back of your eye receives. Lowered lids mean less light and easier interpretation. Lowering the lids also affects the surface of the eye, changing the front of the eye and altering the eye's focus.

But squinting is given a bad name because it is associated with poor vision and the straining of the eyes to see better.

What would happen if you partially closed your lids without straining to see better? You would change your sight, making it more or less blurry. If it was less blurry, you could gradually open your eyes slightly more and see if you can retain that improved focus.

My recent exploration of the eyes has given me a much greater appreciation of the squint and it's cousin, the blink. During and after a blink I can often make out letters on the chart that I could not with open, staring eyes. The fluctuation in the front of my eye has given me more information about the shape, allowing recognition when it eluded me before.

When in doubt about a bit of text, blink more and relax.

These are a few of the things I have found to be helpful. Please use what I've said as a springboard for ideas of exercises that might help your own eyes. Do a couple of clock rotations. Add a finger to the nose and a short bobblehead dance while focusing on the horizon, and you have the beginning of an individualized exercise routine (or the newest dance craze if you film yourself) .

MAKING IT REAL

As you can perhaps tell, there is no end to the things we could do to try and help you physically get your eyes more comfortable and improve your sight. But let's add one more thing. Add something real into your eye exercises, something like catching a ball, something like having your eyes track something in the real world without effort, without straining to see it clearly. If we see something in the real world, we typically lock onto it as if our lives would end if we didn't see it clearly. Practicing an open field of vision, still seeing things in the background while focusing in the foreground, allows you to use the whole back of your eye. You may find that, while your central vision is cloudy, areas of your peripheral vision are still quite sharp. Using those areas, allowing your eyes to accommodate their information, can literally change how you see.

12 A Simple Eye Diet

I began this book with the idea of focusing on foods and perhaps adding in a little exercise. Hopefully you've already gotten the picture that the problem for most eyes is more likely to be blood flow and fluid flow within the eye than what's going into your stomach. No amount of good food is going to get the nutrients where they need to go if you don't change the way your eye moves and functions. Once you've got an exercise routine for your eyes to improve that flow then what you eat does matter.

Diet makes a difference, but we don't have a diet specifically for the eyes. People eating just for their eyes will find themselves frustrated by the lack of studies.

We know that eating enough calories by itself makes a difference. The muscles of the eye have the highest density of energy production of anywhere in the body.[clxx] So they need calories and oxygen to move all the time.

SAD DIET CHOICES

As we spread our Standard American Diet (SAD) around the world, it's no surprise that eyesight is failing. We don't have the human studies, but fat rats have bad eyes.[clxxi]

Compare eyesight problems today to scurvy hundreds of years ago.[clxxii] Scurvy was found to be treated by the vitamin

C in limes, which got the British navy ridiculed as "Limies." But soldiers were still dying of scurvy in the Civil War because the way they prepared their greens destroyed all the vitamin C.[clxxiii] The extent of the problem wasn't acknowledged or dealt with properly.

Even today, when we know that vitamin C helps prevent eye degeneration, it's not commonly prescribed. We know that it is absorbed and can be found in the front of the eye the day after it is taken.[clxxiv] It is likely many other substances profoundly affect the eye. But we're not going to see studies to find out what they are as long as the majority of eye doctors cling to the idea that eye health is genetic.

As we enter a new age of global blindness, we need to refocus our diets onto whole foods. Not just because of the known health benefits, because of those - like avoiding blindness - we are just now starting to understand.

VITAMIN A

Let's take a moment to return to basics. What vitamin is best for your eyes? That's right, vitamin A, eat your carrots. Deficiency in vitamin A can cause blindness. An excess of vitamin A may help prevent eye deterioration.[clxxv] Vitamin A from food can prevent cataracts, glaucoma, and macular degeneration.[clxxvi] So how much talk about vitamin A levels and supplementation is happening in countries with epidemic nearsightedness? None..

How do we get vitamin A? The safest way is not from the straight vitamin (which can build up in the liver when mega-doses are taken) but from those pre-vitamin compounds called beta-carotenes. It's in all those orange and dark green leafy vegetables at the front of the grocery store. The beta carotenes are so safe that if you overdose on them you literally turn orange before anything bad happens to your body organs. It's called carotenemia and it scares doctors because it looks like hepatitis. But other than the orange color, it doesn't seem to do much harm.

Before we all start drinking far too much carrot juice, if you check our best estimates of fruit and vegetable intakes, Asian countries rank highest in the world.[clxxvii] They get the most fruits and vegetables yet they also have the highest rates of nearsightedness. So the issue may be that the fruits and vegetables aren't getting where they need to go, or it may be that the younger Asian population is eating a much different, much lower vegetable diet. We don't have more detailed information to find out for sure, and the issue is confused by poverty, health education, etc.

In a study about whether eating more high vitamin A containing foods would be protective against night blindness in the U.S., researchers found that it didn't make any difference. But that study suffered from the lack of any control group. Women who already had night blindness were far more likely to be eating more carrots. They knew they had a problem and were trying to help themselves.[clxxviii] But it threw off the study trying to see if vitamin A intake was protective against night blindness. (Before we feel bad for these women possibly wasting their time, they were also lowering their risk of certain cancers by as much as half by eating those same carrots.[clxxix])

So instead of a clear picture of something as basic as vitamin A being helpful for the eyes, we're left with the feeling that it might not help that much. It does, but only if the body can get the Vitamin A where it needs to go.

AREDS AND AREDS 2

The most comprehensive study ever done on the eyes

was one called the Age-Related Eye Disease Study (AREDS) which focused on preventing macular degeneration. Researchers found that taking a simple supplement (copper, C, E, Zinc, and beta-carotene) slowed the progression of the disease. Encouraged, they added several more things that seemed to be helpful in smaller diet studies and started AREDS 2.

But it turns out that when you add in a few bits of food as a dry capsule it doesn't perform as well as eating the diet that contains the food. The researchers declared AREDS2 a failure (though the eye supplement industry seems to think it was a success) and moved on to trying to find other bits of food they could add to dry capsules in the hopes that they could still make a difference.

If you're someone with the rare genetically caused version of macular degeneration, you may not benefit from the basic AREDS supplements even if you don't yet have any symptoms. Supplementing relatives of people with that rare form of macular degeneration didn't make any difference in the back of their eyes.[clxxx] Now, these were older people, so they possibly had some deterioration of their eye as well. But the point is that the supplements didn't translate into benefit for them even before they showed any macular degeneration symptoms.

So yes, taking vitamin C, E, zinc, beta-carotene and copper will slow down your progression of macular eye disease by about 25%.[clxxxi] But adding lutein, zeoxanthin, and omega 3 fatty acids as a pill didn't make any difference.[clxxxii] We need to move away from supplements to actual food.

PILLS FOR CATARACTS?

Just because macular degeneration isn't helped much by supplements doesn't mean we aren't trying to cure other eye problems like cataracts with supplements. Cataracts are basically the oxidation of the lens, which can be mimicked by cooking the lens[clxxxiii] (just like a clear egg white becomes cloudy). How cataracts form when they do is still a mystery, though I already put in my two cents about a possible breakdown of that three-named mystery canal being involved.

Miracle supplements like N-acetylcarnosine (NAC) or Lanosterol are really good for animal eyes and may help healthy human eyes. But they may not help diseased eyes. NAC can reverse the cloudy front of a lens (cataract) in a dog's eye,[clxxxiv] but it hasn't been through big human trials[clxxxv] (and there's controversy if it really helps all dogs). Lanosterol is a waxy substance like lanolin, and it clears up cataracts in a test tube, but there's some question about how to get it into the eye by taking it orally (it was injected in the animal studies).[clxxxvi]. Both supplements are sold for dogs, and NAC is sold for humans. If we are to use the reviews as any measure of success (and these are not studies, because reviews can be faked) then about half of those responding got some benefit. That would be in the range of what we would expect, with the other half of those trying the eye drops not having enough blood flow or inner eye transport to get the formulations where they need to go in the eye.

SUPPLEMENTS IN GENERAL

Many of you want to know about your favorite pill, and whether that will make all the difference in your condition. Just as NAC might help with some cataracts, forskolin may help with glaucoma. CoQ10 and melatonin may help a range of eye problems by giving the muscles of the eye more energy. Bilberry may help with computer screen fatigue. Hyaluronic acid may help with dry eyes. Turmeric may help with retinitis pigmentosa.[clxxxvii]

But before you fill up a shopping bag with things for your eye, remember that the issue is more likely to be blood flow than vitamin deficiency. Yes, try those supplements that may help you, but don't rely on them, and if they aren't successful realize that they are likely not getting where they need to go.

FOOD OVER PILLS

So instead of capsules, people with eye diseases have to eat the right diet. By flooding the system with good food, the bare minimum may reach the eyes. For people with high blood sugar, a Mediterranean diet, more fiber, more fish, and fewer calories helps protect their eyes.[clxxxviii] For people with macular degeneration, stopping smoking, a Mediterranean diet, more fish,[clxxxix] and more exercise helps prevent progression.

WHAT IS THE MEDITERRANEAN DIET?

When we talk about a diet, most of us want to know what to eat. But what we're talking about is as much a lifestyle as what you put in your mouth. Here is the description of "the" Mediterranean diet from the Mayo Clinic:

"The Mediterranean diet emphasizes:

Eating primarily plant-based foods, such as fruits and vegetables, whole grains, legumes and nuts
Replacing butter with healthy fats such as olive oil and canola oil

Using herbs and spices instead of salt to flavor foods
Limiting red meat to no more than a few times a
month
Eating fish and poultry at least twice a week
Enjoying meals with family and friends
Drinking red wine in moderation (optional)
Getting plenty of exercise"[cxc]

Notice that the description sounds a lot more crunchy feely than the average doctor's prescription. That's because we're talking about a way of living, not a menu.

We can make some guesses about which foods might specifically be helpful or harmful to aging eyes. Adding fish oil into a mouse's diet helps with eye degeneration.[cxci] Adding fish oil into a human diet decreases dry eyes.[cxcii][cxciii] Feeding mice a high sugar diet made eye degeneration worse.[cxciv] A high sugar diet in human adults results in poorer blood flow in the eyes, regardless of age.[cxcv] The negative results of a high sugar diet on our human eye health only increases with age.[cxcvi]

The deficiency of the supplement compounds in a person's eyes may be a symptom of the disease rather than the cause of macular degeneration. So adding them into a sick person's diet does little good.[cxcvii] They may still benefit from a full dietary change, and we know that the Mediterranean diet may slow their vision loss by as much as 20%.[cxcviii] Will additional supplements help? We don't know beyond the very basics of C, E, zinc and beta-carotene (now switched in many formulas to lutein and xanthine for smokers' benefit). It is possible that the supplements the people with macular degeneration take are being absorbed, but being redirected from the eye into the brain first, where they may slow dementia.[cxcix]

VEGETABLES

Many of you picked up this book specifically for the purpose of finding out what one thing you should eat for your eyes.

In a word, vegetables.

Green, leafy vegetables contain lutein, zeaxanthin, and mesozeaxanthin, the macular carotenoids, building blocks of the back of your eyes. They are literally the stuff your eyes are burning through right now as you try to see these words clearly. Yep, right now you're burning through that lettuce slice or kale chunk. Haven't had any of those recently? Then guess what? You're short, a little deficient. Is it any wonder that your eyes aren't doing great? Even if your eyes are in great shape and see perfectly, those same carotenoids can help you recover from today's glare or strain from seeing.[cc] Green leafy vegetables, even in capsule form, improve healthy eyes in study after study.[cci] They literally thicken the back of your eye, help you with glare, and speed your reaction times.[ccii] A person only needs about 13 milligrams of them for the maximum benefit (more doesn't help as much).[cciii]

We are talking about orange substances: lutein, zeaxanthin, β-carotene and lycopene. These are all found in carrots. But when you try to feed them in high quantities to monkeys, you don't get more of them in the one area of the eye you want them. In other words, more doesn't make you better.[cciv] We do know that not enough can make you worse, increasing the risk of at least cataracts.

So if you're young and relatively healthy, green leafy vegetables are all you need to add in sufficient quantities to improve your eyes. But by the time you have macular degeneration, you may get the stuff you need into your blood stream without it ever reaching your eyes.

Taking larger food level amounts daily, as broccoli, spinach or eggs (the orange part) can lower the risk of cataracts (20%) and macular degeneration (40%).[ccv] But no one is doing large scale studies of the population to see if more will be helpful.[ccvi]

My prediction is that more isn't going to help, and even large amounts may not help people with severe eye diseases because the necessary blood and lymph flow isn't happening within their eyes.

GOOD FATS

If you want to add one more thing to eat with your vegetables, try a good fat. We've known since 1963 that switching from animal fat to unsaturated fat may help with diabetic eyes.[ccvii] We've known since 1965 that essential fatty acid deficiency can negatively affect the eye.[ccviii] So make the switch to olive or coconut oil, and stop buying bargain margarine.

BLOOD FLOW

Whether you add vegetables and good fats or go the whole Mediterranean lifestyle (good for you!) those nutrients have to reach the eye to be helpful. One of the biggest issues with studies of older people with eye problems is that even if you feed them the right capsules their eyes aren't getting the nutrients they need. Things like dry eye, diabetes, and hardening of the arteries is keeping the blood with those nutrients from reaching the inside of the eye.

We know that blood flow affects the eyes because high

cholesterol levels increase the risk of eye disease.[ccix] High sugar levels (diabetes) also raised the risk.[ccx] Both sugar and fat in the arteries slows their ability to get nutrients to the eye. When the nutrients do get there, they fill up the back of the eye first.[ccxi] So the front of the eye, which does all the focusing, is the last place to receive those nutrients. The problem is that the people who need the nutrients aren't getting them where they need to go. Remember, even the best diet is secondary to your daily working plan to gently get your eyes flowing more.

ERASING FALSE BOUNDARIES

We need more studies that show benefit of diet for the "non-permanent" symptoms of eye strain. Something as simple as adding mandarin orange yogurt into a person's diet can significantly improve the symptoms of allergic eyes.[ccxii] A dozen more studies like that would help us figure out which aspects of the Mediterranean diet are the most helpful (I suspect it might be the three hour, cell phone free meal times).

13 How Do I Fix My eyes?

The journey from theory to practice is hardest when there is no known path. We do not have huge studies on how to improve your eyesight. What we have is an ongoing, fifty year global study on how to destroy eyesight over a couple of generations.

The current state of the art medical nearsightedness prevention involves a lifelong prescription to one of several drugs that paralyze the contracting muscles of the eye. The drugs do help prevent progression, but don't improve the eyes. All the other conventional interventions, contacts, and corrective lenses, are less effective at preventing the progression of nearsightedness than the drugs. So we have drugs that slow the progression, but nothing makes it better, and everything else is worse at slowing it down. That's as good as it gets within the conventional model of eyecare.[ccxiii]

Surely, given the state of the standard model, eye doctors would be looking around for alternative solutions? A few are, dubbing themselves Behavioral Optometrists and helping patients alter their vision using a combination of exercises and different lenses.[ccxiv] But they are very quiet and very much on the fringe as the memory of Dr. Bates is still very much with us.

Other doctors are quietly building on the idea of exercises possibly helping. Remarkably, they note, short term eye exercises seem to help progressive nearsighted individuals. But there is no follow-up, no larger idea that possibly the whole framework of inevitable eye deterioration is flawed.[ccxv] Still, their experiments can give some guidance for individuals who want to try exercises on their own.[ccxvi]

WHAT ARE WE TRYING TO FIX?

At the end of the day the "gold standard" of eye health for most of us is whether we can read letters on a chart. Can we talk about these eye charts?

Is practicing how to decipher lines of blurry text somehow cheating? Am I ruining the test by practicing it at home? Or, like any test, does my practicing likely improve my ability to perform the test?

In the last twenty years I've only taken my eye exam a dozen times, and I've had an optometrist tell me I couldn't do what I was trying to do. I remember giving my son timed math tests. The first dozen times he was timed, he panicked. His scores were bad because he was nervous about the test. My son knew the material. But because the testing model was unfamiliar, he panicked. If we had based his math ability on the first dozen tests, he would have been placed several grades below his real ability. Can you imagine what would have happened if I'd told my son he "Just couldn't do it?" It's incredible to me that a test that I can see might be flawed has completely escaped my notice all these years.

In our lives, how often do we take time to puzzle out blurry black and white text? I don't. I just put on my glasses. But if I practice recognizing black and white shapes, is there a downside? The only life situation I can see that being an issue in is if I want to read a faraway sign without my glasses. Currently I push back on my eyelid to shorten my eye and bring it into focus. I definitely wouldn't do that while driving. So there is no "real world" downside to me or you practicing reading blurry letters.

What about me "cheating" and practicing for my eye test? Am I going to end up with the wrong lenses? Well, every time I've ever gone in to see my optometrist we end the appointment with him putting my old prescription in place and then giving me the choice of slight variations. I'm pretty sure the rest of the exam is secondary to this final step. The general testing is just to make sure my eyes haven't "gone south" horribly in the last year. So, other than disrupting my optometrist's expectation that my eyes will always deteriorate, there's no real downside to me improving my ability to read his eye charts and getting a slightly different prescription.

Perhaps we should also ask ourselves how valid these office eye tests really are? Doing medical tests in the doctor's office always makes patients nervous. It doesn't affect something like the chemicals in a blood test, but it can affect things like blood pressure. For blood pressure, we no longer recommend using office tests because the nervous elevation in blood pressure can give invalid results. It's called "white coat syndrome" and can lead to the wrong diagnosis. Patients are now told to do their blood pressures at home, which gives a more realistic idea of their true daily blood pressures.

If blood pressure is not valid in the doctor's office, is the pressure of the eye, which is directly related to blood pressure? I wonder if any patients are being treated for glaucoma when they really have white coat syndrome. And that same anxiety is likely to affect the tension of the muscles inside the eye, making it unlikely that my nervous eye exam is entirely representative of my daily sight.

GO OUTSIDE

If we're looking at the simplest model of improving your eyes, researchers now recommend going outside. The combination of distance viewing and bright light cuts nearsighted progression by about half in most studies.

Ah, but I live in Maine, where there are days when being outside really isn't a great option. Even if I went outside, I doubt I could see much or get much sunlight with all the swirling snow.

If we believe the chicken studies, all I need is an indoor light box, which replicates the light of the sun. The least nearsightedness happened when the chickens were exposed to five hours of bright light a day. Ten hours was worse, so more is not better. To be fair, the best results for nearsightedness happened when the chickens were given a minute of bright light and a minutes of darkness. But that sounds like a nightmare of slow strobe light existence. So I'll take the two-thirds reduction in nearsightedness that five hours of bright light gives me.

20/20/20

You would think that we'd be changing directions in the face of a global pandemic. Maybe rethinking our outlook on screen time at least. But the American Academy of Ophthalmology continues to tell us that, no matter how much we do, "Staring at your computer screen, smartphone or other digital devices for long periods won't cause permanent eye damage"[ccxvii]

The American Optometric Association has paid a little

more attention. They instituted a 20/20/20 rule, which says that for every twenty minutes of screen time you should look twenty feet away for twenty seconds.[ccxviii] Since officially eye exercises still don't help anyone and screen time won't hurt your eyes, where did this rule come from? Surely a major push by one of the two major eye doctor groups would be based on medical research?

There are no studies on medline with any mention of 20/20/20 in them. So I went looking elsewhere for the eye improving benefits of this particular regime. As far as I can tell, there is no scientific justification for this particular set of instructions. Instead of studies on how to reverse the pandemic, we've got a marketing soundbite.

A study done in Nepal found that young people who spent more than two hours at a time looking at a screen almost all had vision problems, and that those vision problems improved if they took lots of breaks.[ccxix] But nothing about 20/20/20. Another study in Saudi Arabia found that -surprise- students who used screens all day tended to have eye problems.[ccxx] Again, no specific 20/20/20 rule. In India researchers found a direct connection between, "increased hours of computer use and the symptoms of redness, burning sensation, blurred vision and dry eyes."[ccxxi] Nothing on 20/20/20. Another study from Japan claims it takes less than one second to shift from near to far sight. In that study students were able to shift back and forth quickly, though some of them didn't show full eye relaxation even after two minutes of moving to distance viewing.[ccxxii]

The idea that it takes twenty seconds for your eyes to fully relax into far vision makes no sense at all. Take a moment to look up from the page and focus on something far away. Does it take twenty seconds for your eyes to refocus? If we think about hunter-gatherer cultures, taking twenty seconds to see far away would lead to starvation or sudden, painful death (a cheetah can cover a third of a mile in twenty seconds, with many other predators not far behind). Children can change from near to far vision in a fraction of a second. So 20/20/20 is just good marketing without any science behind it.

HOW STRAIN LEADS TO DAMAGE

Sure, too much screen time can lead to annoying symptoms, but no permanent damage, right? Well, not at first. Let's spell out how this works. Your eye needs oxygen. The front of your eye needs nutrients to function. Oxygen the eye can get when your eye is open (and moist), but nutrients it only gets when you blink. When you are reading, even this book, your blink rate drops.[ccxxiii] But when you're reading on a screen, you have fewer complete blinks as well.[ccxxiv] Your eyes don't completely close viewing a screen, which means that the nutrients your eye needs don't get to where they need to go.

EXERCISE: SQUINTING

Take a moment to partially close your eyelids with me. Still see the screen or book? Yep, the part of your eye you're using to see, the part that needs nutrients the most, isn't getting those nutrients as much when you read all day. It's much worse when you read on a screen because very few of your blinks cover this overused area.

Depriving your eyes over years of necessary nutrition can lead to permanent damage, despite the assurances of official eye doctor groups. How do I know? Because we're engaged in the largest eye experiment in human history and that's exactly what's happening all over the world.

So how do you begin to fix your eyes? It doesn't start with changing your diet. It starts with changing how much of your diet reaches your eyes. In most cases people are eating enough of what they need, but they don't have decent blood and fluid flow in their eyes to get it to starved tissues.

A REALISTIC PROMISE TO YOURSELF

Rather than rely on a gimmick without any evidence (20/20/20), let's make a deal. Every time your eyes get tired, rest them for a few seconds. If you're falling asleep, tighten them to keep yourself awake rather than drifting off. But don't think that day-in, day-out eye irritation, pain, and fatigue doesn't have a cost.

You can offset that deterioration immediately, as soon it happens, by giving your eyes a break. Think of eye irritation as the eye's version of panting. If you're panting hard enough when you run, you have to slow down. The eye is just signaling the same situation. It's time to take a little mini-break, a couple of long blinks.

Beyond those basic nutritional eye breaks built in throughout your waking day, you need to tailor your own routine. You want to improve your eyes without exhausting yourself. We're not talking about physical exhaustion but exhausting your willpower. It's fine to do binges of eye movement and stretches, but it's going to be the day-to-day changes you can keep doing that will really make the difference.

Chances are that your eyes got where they are after decades. So reversing that process is going to take months if not a few years even if you find the perfect mix of exercises.

For me sticking to improving my eyes means "playing" with my eyes, doing very short bursts of different exercises, exploring different options, and not establishing a routine that I have to do. I need to have fun with it, or I won't keep doing it. (Right now I'm typing wearing my junior high school glasses with a pirate eyepatch over my right eye in an effort to get my left eye back to where it was in junior high. Arrgh, matey!)

For some of you it will be the opposite. You want to set up a daily routine and keep to it. Hopefully you'll get so used to it that it becomes an unconscious habit and you forget there was a time you didn't do it

ASSESS WHERE YOU ARE

I cannot predict what state your eyes are in, and what your goals might be. Some of you want to preserve a little sight, while others might be trying to achieve superhumanly far vision. So I want to give you the basics for how to achieve your goals, whatever they may be.

MEASURE WHAT YOU WANT TO CHANGE

First, you need to have a way to measure progress. Getting a long distance chart and a near vision chart are the first two steps. If you really can't see the far vision chart, start by modifying the distance you are from the chart. Maybe you can only read the big letter E at three feet, or maybe you can read it at three hundred feet (hint, if that is the case shrink the text size down to a fraction of its original size until it fits into your space - unless you happen to have a three hundred foot room handy). The goal of the charts isn't to have the perfect set-up. It's to have a consistent set-up that allows you to measure yourself against a set of markers that don't change day-to-day. If you can tell you're making progress, that's all that matters.

WHAT CAN YOU DO EASILY… FOR THE REST OF YOUR LIFE?

Next, what should you do to improve your eyes? Well, what will you do easily every day without resentment to improve your eyes? Sure, I could say no screen time for a year and throw away your glasses. Or spend the next six months staring in deep relaxation at the sea horizon in Bali while taking enormously deep breaths, eating a vegan Mediterranean diet, and blinking sixty times a minute. But chances are some of you now want to throw this book across the room. We all have lives and obligations.

Instead of the eye boot camp model, let's go for moderate steps. Moderate your screen time (geez, I hate this one already). Batch your phone browsing to once every fifteen minutes, thirty minutes, or even once an hour. (This one is easier for me, because I'm a phone flake). Start not using your corrective lenses for longer periods of the day. If you have them, use yellow/computer or at least different lenses for your screens.

SET LOW, ACHIEVABLE GOALS

How many exercises you want to bring into your routine depends on your goals. I recommend a bar so low you think it's really possible.

My goal when I started this book was to be able to read the labels on groceries again without taking my glasses on and off in the grocery store. It was an impossible goal, one my optometrist told me could never happen. I achieved that goal in three weeks, with minimal effort.

So now my more recent goal is to even out my eyes, so that my "bad" left eye can see as well as my good right eye for near vision at least. That's why right now I look like pirate Jack with my right eye patch. My left eye is slowly getting used to having to carry more of the load.

How did I achieve my initial label reading goal? It was deceptively simple. In the first couple of experiments I did with my eyes, I realized that the amount of light reflecting off the letters of the groceries I was viewing made a great deal of difference. Rather than accepting what I was and wasn't seeing, I began to try and see differently. Not with tension or strain, but by moving my eyes around, trying to see from different angles. I realized after a couple of days that my right eye could see more clearly for near vision than my left. Once I focused on just the right eye, and "gave it permission" (there isn't any other way to describe it), my right eye began to focus better on smaller and smaller print. Rather than telling my right eye that it was old, and couldn't see, I let my right eye tell me what it could see.

In the grocery store, I now tilt the groceries up to the light before trying to see them, I allow myself space to view them without getting nervous (tension) or frustrated, and I know that I can read the smaller print under the right conditions. The combination means that I'm reading labels without thinking consciously about it. My first experience of this was realizing with a start that I hadn't taken off my glasses the whole time I'd been in the store. It's just become part of who I am again. Although I have to say label text sizes can be really small and in yellow print, so give yourself permission rather than spending a half hour trying to make out some candy bar wrapper.

Let's talk about my initial goal and put it into context. I didn't really have time to alter the strength of my eyes before I could see labels again. My optometrist may say that my focusing ability has not changed objectively by his measurements. So my eyes may not be officially improved.

But I can see better. I've learned to use my eyes more effectively, found a way around whatever short comings old age has given me.

Objectively, I see better. No, I may not do better on my yearly eye test, but I'm doing better in my life.

Just like any other test given to any schoolchild on any day of the school year, my eye test only gives a snapshot of one aspect of my ability. I now realize that conditions like background lighting, eye fatigue, and my attitude can affect how well my eyes perform.

For my second goal, I'm working with my weaker left eye. Since my goal is to be able to use that left eye as well as my right, I've been reading with my right eye closed, both with and without glasses. Not obsessively, just as it occurs to me. For example, I had my right eye closed for part of this sentence when I was editing the book.

What I've already noticed is that my near vision for my left, which was almost non-existent, has at least entered onto the near-vision chart at the upper end. Surprisingly, I've also noticed that my distance vision for my left eye seems clearer as well. It's hard to tell, because the big "E" seems less blurry.

What I've started doing recently with the distance eye chart is halving the distance so I can read more letters rather than squinting (straining tension) at letters I cannot read. I'm roughly 20/350 so reading the top line (20/200) at half distance means I'm roughly working at my limit. Remember, I see at twenty feet what other people can see at three hundred and fifty feet without glasses. So cutting my distance in half gives me a fighting chance to see the top of the board. I haven't yet seen much improvement in my distance vision at ten feet away so I'm suspicious my eyes learned to strain to see in the distance really well and it will take time for me to retrain myself.

If Dr. Bates was right, and strain affects sight, then all I've been doing by straining at the board from ten feet away is hurting my eyes every day. In reality, all eye doctors agree that eye strain occurs. It's their bread-and-butter. Don't want eye strain? Buy these glasses or get this surgery. The only disagreement they have with Bates (one I think Bates is winning) is whether daily eye strain over decades can cause permanent eye damage.

When I tried halving my distance, I can see the top of the distance charts. Then I backed up to my normal blurry viewing distance and the strangest thing happened. I turned my head with just my left eye open and saw the top E perfectly. Then a little voice in my head (some past teacher or doctor?) told me, "No, you can't read that," and the line went blurry.

It was the strangest experience. Someone in the last forty years might well have said that to me. I can easily picture an eye doctor noticing the time and hurrying me along. Rather than "Is this better?" she might have told me I couldn't read the line because I was pausing too long. Since I try to be a perfect patient (and fail) I may have taken it to heart. It's hard to read so I just can't read it.

But what I've already discovered about myself is that with a little time and creativity, I can read that. In a few moments with the distance letters at half the distance, my right eye can read the second line. Why can't it read the second line on my newer, less familiar distance eye chart? The line is hard to make out, and when it's hard to make out I've learned to stop trying.

DON'T GET FANATICAL

In contrast to the doctors, individuals who have found their own way to better eyesight tend to be militant in their stance. Defensive statements, angry arguments with optometrists, these are the norm. Yes, these particular patients were able to get better (one well-known online subject used progressively weaker lenses over time to retrain his eyes)[ccxxv] But that is because of their high level of dedication and focus on the issue. Think of them as the equivalent to any exercise or weight loss testimonial. While it's true that eating just kale is truly a weight loss miracle, very few of us will likely have the same results without the same level of fanatical dedication.

SETTING UP YOUR GOALS

My goals are both relatively modest and officially impossible. I know that I can achieve them. Rather than deciding that you'll have perfect vision in two weeks I'd recommend trying to not have your eyes hurt as much at the end of the day. Perhaps try to see things with less blurriness, or simply explore what vision you have to see what you can maximize for yourself.

Remember that you will improve your sight as you put attention toward seeing better. That improvement may not translate in an optometrist's office or into eyeglass changes, but it will be tangible and fairly immediate as part of your daily experience.

I was startled at a stoplight recently. Looking above the edge of my glasses, I could fuzzily make out the letters indicating a left turn only signal. For the last several decades if you'd asked me if that was possible, I would have told you no. I needed my glasses to read all road signage. But, while my glasses haven't changed (yet?) my brain's ability to interpret what I'm seeing blurrily has improved.

HERE ARE THE STEPS FOR FIXING YOUR EYES:

1) Choose a very reasonable, achievable short-term goal (my eyes will be less tired, hurt less, etc.)

2) Set up a way to measure your eyesight that is consistent for you.

3) Begin doing the minimum you think is necessary to achieve your short-term goal.

4) Increase what you're doing only if your short-term goal isn't achieved within a reasonable (non-frustrating) period of time.

5) Once your short-term goal is achieved, set another, easily achievable short-term goal.

6) Do the bare minimum required to achieve each goal, knowing that every day you are improving by putting even a little attention toward that goal.

7) Be prepared to "fall off the wagon" and forget to do the work toward your goals. Forgive yourself now, love yourself despite it, and make it easier for yourself by altering the goal to fit your life. You aren't running a marathon, you're living a life. Every little bit helps.

Do we look for studies on whether practicing the piano helps? Sight is not unique among the senses. It, too, can be improved with practice.
-C. J. Maloney

ABOUT THE AUTHOR

There is no better way to thank God for your sight than by giving a helping hand to someone in the dark.-Helen Keller

Of all Christopher Maloney's possessions, he has often prized his glasses the most. An avid rule follower, he wore his glasses nonstop during every waking hour for decades. Different glasses were shattered over time, causing him pain and a sense of loss comparable to losing a pet. Since writing this book, he has started using his glasses less and seeing more. Dr. Maloney had colon cancer in 2015, so he already follows a diet far more restrictive than recommended here. He has noticed no weight loss, but a loss of two belt loops of belly fat since starting. His books are available at naturopathicmaine.com and chrisjlmaloney.com.

Thanks for reading! If you enjoyed the book, please review it. Other readers can only find the book if it has enough reviews. Thanks!

---

[i] https://www.ncbi.nlm.nih.gov/pubmed/15989747

[ii] https://www.medicalnewstoday.com/articles/317663.php

[iii] https://www.ncbi.nlm.nih.gov/pubmed/28384718

[iv] https://www.ncbi.nlm.nih.gov/pubmed/1937488

[v] https://www.ncbi.nlm.nih.gov/pmc/articles/PMC4779297/

[vi] https://www.ncbi.nlm.nih.gov/pubmed/27898441

[vii] http://www.thelancet.com/journals/lancet/article/PIIS0140-6736(12)60272-4/abstract

[viii] http://www.who.int/blindness/causes/MyopiaReportforWeb.pdf

[ix] https://www.ncbi.nlm.nih.gov/pubmed/22161388

[x] https://www.cnn.com/2015/04/05/asia/myopia-east-asia/index.html

[xi] https://www.ncbi.nlm.nih.gov/pubmed/26875007

[xii] https://www.ncbi.nlm.nih.gov/pubmed/28980750

[xiii] http://onlinelibrary.wiley.com/doi/10.1111/j.1600-0420.2005.00352.x/pdf

[xiv] http://www.aaojournal.org/article/S0161-6420(16)00025-7/fulltext

[xv] https://www.sciencedirect.com/science/article/pii/S0161642016000257

[xvi] https://www.ncbi.nlm.nih.gov/pubmed/8153707

[xvii] https://www.ncbi.nlm.nih.gov/pubmed/28733687

[xviii] https://www.sciencedirect.com/science/article/pii/004269899400233C

[xix] https://www.ncbi.nlm.nih.gov/pubmed/27537606

[xx] https://www.ncbi.nlm.nih.gov/pubmed/22167095

[xxi] http://hyperphysics.phy-astr.gsu.edu/hbase/vision/eyescal.html

[xxii] https://www.aao.org/eye-health/glasses-contacts-list

[xxiii] https://www.ncbi.nlm.nih.gov/pubmed/12022898

[xxiv] https://www.ncbi.nlm.nih.gov/pubmed/29242183

[xxv] https://youtu.be/vJG698U2Mvo

[xxvi] https://en.wikipedia.org/wiki/Fovea_centralis

[xxvii] http://fs.aoa.org/optometry-archives/optometry-timeline.html

[xxviii] http://fs.aoa.org/optometry-archives/optometry-timeline.html

[xxix] https://archive.org/stream/optometryontrial00byro/optometryontrial00byro_djvu.txt

[xxx] http://fs.aoa.org/optometry-archives/optometry-timeline.html

[xxxi] https://www.ncbi.nlm.nih.gov/pubmed/23952133

[xxxii] https://www.ncbi.nlm.nih.gov/pubmed/22373170

[xxxiii] https://www.ncbi.nlm.nih.gov/pmc/articles/PMC510603/?page=1

[xxxiv] https://www.aao.org/about/history

[xxxv] https://www.ncbi.nlm.nih.gov/pubmed/28870179

[xxxvi] https://www.ncbi.nlm.nih.gov/pubmed/22161388

[xxxvii] https://books.google.com/books?id=MilnrDgQiwgC&pg=PA372-IA64&lpg=PA372-IA64&dq=William+H.+Bates+obituary+NYT&source=bl&ots=uJC2LOsAzb&sig=Len-Jp0boi1KsmS7Ct3v9jcwr3s&hl=en&sa=X&ved=0ahUKEwjS-qPZseTYAhVqja0KHaknBmEQ6AEIVjAJ#v=onepage&q=William%20H.%20Bates%20obituary%20NYT&f=false

[xxxviii] https://www.iblindness.org/ebooks/perfect-sight-without-glasses/

[xxxix] https://www.iblindness.org/ebooks/perfect-sight-without-glasses/ch-1-introductory/

xl https://www.iblindness.org/ebooks/perfect-sight-without-glasses/ch-1-introductory/

xli https://en.wikipedia.org/wiki/Herman_Snellen

xlii https://www.iblindness.org/ebooks/perfect-sight-without-glasses/ch-1-introductory/

xliii https://www.ncbi.nlm.nih.gov/pubmed/19033886

xliv https://www.ncbi.nlm.nih.gov/pubmed/3532811

xlv https://www.ncbi.nlm.nih.gov/pubmed/28923583

xlvi http://self-healing.org/meir-schneider/

xlvii https://www.sciencedirect.com/topics/neuroscience/ciliary-muscle

xlviii https://www.aao.org/bcscsnippetdetail.aspx?id=f38d473f-c836-4fe6-8555-20d34ce19816

xlix https://www.ncbi.nlm.nih.gov/pubmed/28951958

l https://www.ncbi.nlm.nih.gov/pubmed/29386651

li https://www.ncbi.nlm.nih.gov/books/NBK235051/

lii https://www.ncbi.nlm.nih.gov/pubmed/28549092

liii https://www.ncbi.nlm.nih.gov/pubmed/23493295

liv https://www.ncbi.nlm.nih.gov/pubmed/20592235

lv https://www.ncbi.nlm.nih.gov/pubmed/21423141

lvi https://www.ncbi.nlm.nih.gov/pubmed/20447396

lvii http://endmyopia.org/wp-content/uploads/2017/02/Reduction_in_Axial_Length_with_Age__An.3.pdf

lviii https://www.ncbi.nlm.nih.gov/pmc/articles/PMC5697689/

lix https://www.ncbi.nlm.nih.gov/pubmed/29216865

[lx] https://www.lasikmd.com/blog/eye-shapes-affect-vision

[lxi] https://www.ncbi.nlm.nih.gov/pubmed/28671403

[lxii] https://www.ncbi.nlm.nih.gov/pubmed/16360207

[lxiii] https://www.ncbi.nlm.nih.gov/pubmed/28596969

[lxiv] http://www.aoafoundation.org/ohs/hindsight/optometrist-jailed-for-charging-an-exam-fee/

[lxv] https://www.oepf.org/sites/default/files/journals/jbo-volume-2-issue-2/2-2%20trachtman.pdf

[lxvi] http://www.ajo.com/article/0002-9394(46)91035-5/abstract

[lxvii] http://www.ajo.com/article/S0002-9394(47)91862-X/fulltext

[lxviii] https://www.ncbi.nlm.nih.gov/pubmed/7130612

[lxix] https://www.ncbi.nlm.nih.gov/pubmed/15115060

[lxx] https://www.ncbi.nlm.nih.gov/pubmed/3307440

[lxxi] https://www.cnn.com/2015/04/05/asia/myopia-east-asia/index.html

[lxxii] https://www.nature.com/articles/srep28531

[lxxiii] https://www.ncbi.nlm.nih.gov/pubmed/24008929

[lxxiv] https://www.ncbi.nlm.nih.gov/pubmed/12427060

[lxxv] https://www.ncbi.nlm.nih.gov/pubmed/15642811

[lxxvi] https://www.ncbi.nlm.nih.gov/pubmed/24179885

[lxxvii] https://www.ncbi.nlm.nih.gov/pmc/articles/PMC5769202/

[lxxviii] https://www.ncbi.nlm.nih.gov/pubmed/29191783

[lxxix] https://www.ncbi.nlm.nih.gov/pmc/articles/PMC3665208/

[lxxx] https://www.ncbi.nlm.nih.gov/pubmed/28494063

[lxxxi] http://www.nejm.org/doi/full/10.1056/NEJMra1012354

[lxxxii] https://www.ncbi.nlm.nih.gov/pubmed/20207005

[lxxxiii] https://www.ncbi.nlm.nih.gov/pmc/articles/PMC3469316/#R133

[lxxxiv] https://www.ncbi.nlm.nih.gov/pubmed/3307440

[lxxxv] http://biology.anu.edu.au/epidemic-myopia-east-and-southeast-asia

[lxxxvi] https://www.cnn.com/2015/04/05/asia/myopia-east-asia/index.html

[lxxxvii] https://www.ncbi.nlm.nih.gov/pubmed/27618415

[lxxxviii] https://thediplomat.com/2015/03/the-problem-with-taiwanese-eyes/

[lxxxix] http://www.pointsdevue.com/article/prevalence-and-risk-factors-myopia-among-schoolchildren-chimi-taiwan

[xc] http://onlinelibrary.wiley.com/doi/10.1111/aos.13403/full

[xci] https://www.ncbi.nlm.nih.gov/pubmed/28063778

[xcii] https://www.ncbi.nlm.nih.gov/pubmed/27618415

[xciii] https://www.ncbi.nlm.nih.gov/pubmed/28063778

[xciv] https://sciencing.com/light-bulbs-not-emit-uv-radiation-15925.html

[xcv] https://www.ncbi.nlm.nih.gov/pubmed/29356366

[xcvi] https://www.ncbi.nlm.nih.gov/pubmed/24928818

[xcvii] https://www.ncbi.nlm.nih.gov/pmc/articles/PMC5697689/

[xcviii] https://www.ncbi.nlm.nih.gov/pubmed/24950905

[xcix] https://www.ncbi.nlm.nih.gov/pubmed/21917938

[c] https://www.ncbi.nlm.nih.gov/pubmed/29338123

[ci] https://www.ncbi.nlm.nih.gov/pubmed/25698200

cii https://www.aoa.org/patients-and-public/good-vision-throughout-life/adult-vision-19-to-40-years-of-age/adult-vision-41-to-60-years-of-age

ciii https://www.ncbi.nlm.nih.gov/pubmed/29551993

civ https://nei.nih.gov/eyedata/amd

cv https://nei.nih.gov/eyedata/myopia

cvi https://www.ncbi.nlm.nih.gov/pubmed/29607217

cvii https://www.ncbi.nlm.nih.gov/pubmed/25142847

cviii https://www.ncbi.nlm.nih.gov/pubmed/17108845

cix http://www.allaboutvision.com/conditions/presbyopia.htm

cx https://www.ncbi.nlm.nih.gov/pubmed/22440400

cxi http://www.allaboutvision.com/visionsurgery/corneal-inlays-onlays.htm

cxii https://www.ncbi.nlm.nih.gov/pubmed/29577954

cxiii https://www.ncbi.nlm.nih.gov/pubmed/26679984

cxiv https://www.ncbi.nlm.nih.gov/pubmed/24247317

cxv https://www.ncbi.nlm.nih.gov/pmc/articles/PMC2809804/

cxvi https://www.ncbi.nlm.nih.gov/pubmed/8963161/

cxvii http://www.thelancet.com/journals/lancet/article/PIIS0140-6736(12)60272-4/abstract

cxviii https://www.sciencedirect.com/science/article/pii/S0014483510002976

cxix https://www.ncbi.nlm.nih.gov/pmc/articles/PMC1939820/

cxx https://www.ncbi.nlm.nih.gov/pmc/articles/PMC3968930/

cxxi http://www.biometricupdate.com/201508/eyeverify-technology-uses-smartphone-cameras-to-easily-verify-id-by-eye-veins [cxxii] https://www.sciencedirect.com/science/article/pii/S1350946202000083?via%3Dihub

[cxxiii] https://www.ncbi.nlm.nih.gov/pubmed/16488940/

[cxxiv] https://www.ncbi.nlm.nih.gov/pmc/articles/PMC3032230/

[cxxv] http://eyewiki.aao.org/Computational_Fluid_Dynamics_(CFD)_in_Ophthalmology

[cxxvi] https://www.ncbi.nlm.nih.gov/pmc/articles/PMC4274296/

[cxxvii] http://eyewiki.aao.org/Computational_Fluid_Dynamics_(CFD)_in_Ophthalmology

[cxxviii] https://www.ncbi.nlm.nih.gov/pmc/articles/PMC3669488/

[cxxix] https://www.ncbi.nlm.nih.gov/pubmed/29150215

[cxxx] https://www.ncbi.nlm.nih.gov/pmc/articles/PMC5643502/

[cxxxi] http://www.aaojournal.org/article/S0161-6420(14)00433-3/abstract

[cxxxii] https://www.ncbi.nlm.nih.gov/pmc/articles/PMC4535453/

[cxxxiii] https://www.ncbi.nlm.nih.gov/pmc/articles/PMC5496280/

[cxxxiv] https://www.ncbi.nlm.nih.gov/pubmed/28957399

[cxxxv] https://www.ncbi.nlm.nih.gov/pmc/articles/PMC2720680/

[cxxxvi] https://www.ncbi.nlm.nih.gov/pmc/articles/PMC5678323/

[cxxxvii] https://www.ncbi.nlm.nih.gov/pubmed/22324772

[cxxxviii] https://www.ncbi.nlm.nih.gov/pubmed/24133024

[cxxxix] https://www.ncbi.nlm.nih.gov/pmc/articles/PMC5643502/

[cxl] https://wwwnc.cdc.gov/eid/article/23/7/16-1608_article

[cxli] https://www.scientificamerican.com/article/two-eyes-two-views/

cxlii https://www.smithsonianmag.com/science-nature/but-did-you-see-the-gorilla-the-problem-with-inattentional-blindness-17339778/

cxliii https://www.theatlantic.com/health/archive/2014/02/training-your-brain-to-improve-your-vision/283933/

cxliv https://www.waynesburg.edu/docman/70-the-observance-of-the-visual-reaction-time-of-non-athletes-compared-to-athletes/file

cxlv https://www.ncbi.nlm.nih.gov/pmc/articles/PMC4697066/

cxlvi https://www.ncbi.nlm.nih.gov/pubmed/28914003

cxlviicxlvii https://www.aoa.org/patients-and-public/caring-for-your-vision/protecting-your-vision/computer-vision-syndrome

cxlviii https://www.ncbi.nlm.nih.gov/pmc/articles/PMC5532554/

cxlix https://www.youtube.com/watch?v=63tKLX4Zkgo

cl https://www.youtube.com/watch?v=xGMRmoR7GPk

cli https://www.ncbi.nlm.nih.gov/pubmed/29023169

clii https://www.ncbi.nlm.nih.gov/pubmed/27275655

cliii http://onlinelibrary.wiley.com/doi/10.1111/j.1600-0420.2005.00352.x/pdf

cliv http://healthland.time.com/2012/05/07/why-up-to-90-of-asian-schoolchildren-are-nearsighted

clv https://www.ncbi.nlm.nih.gov/pubmed/11149432

clvi https://www.ncbi.nlm.nih.gov/pubmed/12147605

clvii https://www.ncbi.nlm.nih.gov/pubmed/28602573

clviii https://www.sciencedirect.com/science/article/pii/S0014483512002497

clix https://www.ncbi.nlm.nih.gov/pubmed/24179885

clx https://www.ncbi.nlm.nih.gov/pubmed/20207005

clxi https://www.ncbi.nlm.nih.gov/pubmed/9283848

clxii https://www.ncbi.nlm.nih.gov/pubmed/28570621

clxiii https://www.aao.org/eye-health/tips-prevention/vision-training-not-proven-to-make-vision-sharper

clxiv https://www.colorado.edu/physics/phys1230/phys1230_fa01/topic37.html

clxv https://www.improveeyesighthq.com/20-20-vision.html

clxvi https://www.ncbi.nlm.nih.gov/pubmed/26614629

clxvii https://www.ncbi.nlm.nih.gov/pubmed/26578911

clxviii https://www.ncbi.nlm.nih.gov/books/NBK10991/

clxix http://www.davidwebberseeingclearly.com/new-page-1/

clxx https://www.sciencedirect.com/topics/neuroscience/ciliary-muscle

clxxi https://www.ncbi.nlm.nih.gov/pubmed/29075814

clxxii https://news.nationalgeographic.com/2017/01/scurvy-disease-discovery-jonathan-lamb/

clxxiii http://civilwardaybyday.web.unc.edu/nutrition-and-the-war/

clxxiv https://www.ncbi.nlm.nih.gov/pubmed/28693452

clxxv https://www.ncbi.nlm.nih.gov/pmc/articles/PMC2882531/

clxxvi https://www.ncbi.nlm.nih.gov/pubmed/28582804

clxxvii http://bmjopen.bmj.com/content/5/9/e008705?utm_source=TrendMD&utm_medium=cpc&utm_campaign=BMJOp_TrendMD-0

clxxviii https://www.ncbi.nlm.nih.gov/pubmed/10484191

clxxix https://www.ncbi.nlm.nih.gov/pubmed/29100438

clxxx https://www.ncbi.nlm.nih.gov/pubmed/28973076

clxxxi https://www.ncbi.nlm.nih.gov/pmc/articles/PMC3469316/#R13

clxxxii https://web.emmes.com/study/areds2/resources/areds2_press_release_050513.pdf

clxxxiii https://www.ncbi.nlm.nih.gov/pubmed/18547562

clxxxiv https://www.ncbi.nlm.nih.gov/pubmed/15139774

clxxxv https://www.ncbi.nlm.nih.gov/pubmed/12001824

clxxxvi https://www.pbs.org/newshour/science/eye-drops-clear-cataracts

clxxxvii http://www.townsendletter.com/April2018/April2018.html

clxxxviii https://www.ncbi.nlm.nih.gov/pubmed/29324740

clxxxix https://www.ncbi.nlm.nih.gov/pubmed/28153441

cxc https://www.mayoclinic.org/healthy-lifestyle/nutrition-and-healthy-eating/in-depth/mediterranean-diet/art-20047801

cxci https://www.ncbi.nlm.nih.gov/pubmed/28961167

cxcii https://www.ncbi.nlm.nih.gov/pubmed/28371493

cxciii https://www.ncbi.nlm.nih.gov/pubmed/25193932

cxciv https://www.ncbi.nlm.nih.gov/pubmed/28757158

cxcv https://www.ncbi.nlm.nih.gov/pubmed/27756385

cxcvi https://www.ncbi.nlm.nih.gov/pubmed/23531363

cxcvii https://www.ncbi.nlm.nih.gov/pubmed/28756618

cxcviii https://www.ncbi.nlm.nih.gov/pubmed/27825655

cxcix https://www.ncbi.nlm.nih.gov/pubmed/27776568

cc https://www.ncbi.nlm.nih.gov/pubmed/27857944

cci https://www.ncbi.nlm.nih.gov/pubmed/25468896

[ccii] https://www.ncbi.nlm.nih.gov/pmc/articles/PMC5532554/

[cciii] https://www.ncbi.nlm.nih.gov/pubmed/27426932

[cciv] https://www.ncbi.nlm.nih.gov/pubmed/28075370

[ccv] https://www.ncbi.nlm.nih.gov/pubmed/11023002

[ccvi] https://www.ncbi.nlm.nih.gov/pubmed/26042352

[ccvii] https://www.ncbi.nlm.nih.gov/pmc/articles/PMC505868/?page=5

[ccviii] https://www.ncbi.nlm.nih.gov/pubmed/14342243

[ccix] https://www.ncbi.nlm.nih.gov/pubmed/29335418

[ccx] https://www.ncbi.nlm.nih.gov/pubmed/29078839

[ccxi] https://www.ncbi.nlm.nih.gov/pubmed/15656089

[ccxii] https://www.ncbi.nlm.nih.gov/pubmed/28593244

[ccxiii] https://www.ncbi.nlm.nih.gov/pubmed/22161388

[ccxiv] https://my.imatrixbase.com/vision-therapy-pa.com/behavioral-optometry-vision-therapy/introduction-to-dr.-gallop---s-book--looking-differently-at-nearsightedness-and-myopia.html

[ccxv] https://journals.lww.com/optvissci/Fulltext/2009/11000/Accommodative_Training_to_Reduce_Nearwork_Induced.11.aspx

[ccxvi] http://endmyopia.org/wp-content/uploads/2017/08/Accommodative_Training_to_Reduce_Nearwork_Induced.11.pdf

[ccxvii] https://www.aao.org/eye-health/tips-prevention/computer-usage

[ccxviii] https://www.aoa.org/patients-and-public/caring-for-your-vision/protecting-your-vision/computer-vision-syndrome

[ccxix] https://www.ncbi.nlm.nih.gov/pubmed/24172549

[ccxx] https://www.ncbi.nlm.nih.gov/pubmed/29114189

[ccxxi] https://www.ncbi.nlm.nih.gov/pubmed/24761234

[ccxxii] http://onlinelibrary.wiley.com/doi/10.1111/j.1600-0420.2005.00352.x/pdf

[ccxxiii] https://www.ncbi.nlm.nih.gov/pubmed/26517404

[ccxxiv] https://www.ncbi.nlm.nih.gov/pubmed/23538437

[ccxxv] http://endmyopia.org/